C000040182

The
HEALTHY EATING
Handbook

Including essential tips on diet and nutrition; a healthy eating journal;
fat, fibre, vitamin and mineral and calorie counters; and low fat recipes.

The
HEALTHY EATING
Handbook

Including essential tips on diet and nutrition; a healthy eating journal;
fat, fibre, vitamin and mineral and calorie counters; and low fat recipes.

bay books

CONTENTS

FAT, FIBRE & CARBOHYDRATE COUNTER

VITAMIN & MINERAL COUNTER

VITAMINS & OTHER NUTRIENTS

MINERALS

FOOD JOURNAL

FOOD TERMS

THE BENEFITS OF HEALTHY EATING

The food we eat does more than simply fill an empty stomach. Our physical and mental health is directly affected by each and every morsel that passes our lips.

If you want to improve your health, both now and in the future, and the way you look and feel, a healthy lifestyle that includes regular exercise and a balanced diet is the key to achieving this goal. Your dietary habits have a direct effect on your physical and mental health. This isn't surprising when you consider that the foods and drinks you consume actually become part of your body—they are broken down by your digestive system and then absorbed into your cells to provide you with energy or materials for growth, repair and vital bodily processes. So it's true—you are what you eat. And if you don't feed your body all the elements it needs, you won't feel or perform as well as you could.

It's estimated that more than 50 per cent of people in industrialised countries die from nutrition-related diseases (heart disease, stroke, some cancers, diabetes) and many people are also overweight, which can further increase the risk of developing some diseases. This is a sad state of affairs when many of these early deaths could have been prevented by a healthy lifestyle.

Disease isn't only due to bad luck or genetics, it also depends on how well you treat your body. Lifestyle factors play an important role in determining your state of health, which means you can actually play an active role in protecting yourself.

Many people complain of a lack of energy and vitality, and often feel tired and run-down. This is often due to poor dietary habits, which make it more difficult to cope with life's demands, and a stressful environment. By choosing the best foods for your body and by keeping active, you will feel more energetic and protect yourself against disease at the same time.

Some benefits of a healthy lifestyle
- Better mental and physical performance
- A better-looking body
- A better self-image
- Higher energy levels
- A well-functioning immune system
- Lower blood cholesterol levels
- A reduced risk of many diseases
- Attaining a healthy weight without strict dieting

Another good reason to look after your health as you grow older is that people in western societies have never had such a long life-expectancy and good quality of life to look forward to after they retire. Since the start of the 1900s, the average life-expectancy for men and women has increased by more than 20 years. From a relatively young age, we're encouraged to start saving for our retirement, but you should also be investing in your health. Like your income, your health also needs protection as you age, so that when you retire you'll be able to enjoy all the things you missed during full-time employment or parenthood. If you don't have a healthy lifestyle when you're young, you may have to spend more of your hard-earned retirement money on medication, doctors' fees and higher insurance premiums. Unlike investing in the stock market, there's no risk involved in looking after your health.

Although many people regularly take vitamin and mineral supplements, there's little evidence that they give you the same or as many health benefits as a balanced diet. Spend your money on a wide variety of good-quality fresh foods so that you don't need to take supplements, and make time to prepare some of the great-tasting recipes in this book. You'll soon see how easy it is to prepare healthy meals, and you'll wonder why anyone thinks healthy eating isn't enjoyable.

Often healthy, low-fat dishes use more flavoursome ingredients than their high-fat counterparts. Far from being boring or bland, healthy food really does taste great.

WHY ALL THE CONFUSION ABOUT HEALTHY EATING?

Many people are confused about healthy eating because there is so much contradictory information published in newspapers, magazines, books and on the Internet. This information can be written by qualified health professionals and nutrition scientists, or by journalists and business people—who may not have the relevant qualifications.

Although food manufacturers are subject to strict laws preventing them from printing any misleading health claims on their products, other sources of nutrition information are not subject to the same laws, which is a constant source of frustration for health professionals. It is difficult for officials to regulate all the information that is published because there's simply too much information and advertising from so many different sources.

Some people also have a vested interest in telling you that particular diets or supplements produce certain effects because they are trying to sell you these products. Others simply don't know that they haven't researched their information thoroughly enough to be able to give you the whole story.

You need considerable training and background knowledge to be able to interpret the results from scientific studies, and also to decide whether or not the studies have used appropriate methods.

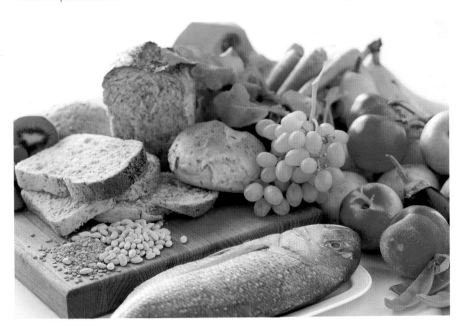

Nutrition science is a young and dynamic science. As more research tools are being developed, we are learning more about the active chemicals in foods and how they affect our health. There are still many exciting new discoveries to be made.

But here's the good news—official science-based recommendations for healthy eating have changed very little over the last 20 years, despite all of the new research findings. For decades the recipe for health has been a diet based on low-fat grain products, legumes, fruits and vegetables, with moderate amounts of lean meat and dairy products. And there's no indication that this message will change.

FOOD ALLERGIES AND INTOLERANCES

WHAT IS A FOOD ALLERGY?

Although many people claim to suffer from allergies to foods or food ingredients, only a very small number of people actually have a true food allergy. A true food allergy happens when the body's immune system overreacts to an otherwise harmless compound in a food or food ingredient, recognising it instead as a foreign substance, like a virus, that needs to be attacked with antibodies.

The compound in the food that stimulates the immune system of allergic people is called an allergen. A single food can contain several allergens, most of which are proteins. A few food-allergic individuals are so sensitive that just touching or even smelling the offending food can cause an allergic reaction. Others must actually eat the food before they get an allergic reaction. Symptoms of food allergies include sneezing, a runny nose, asthma, rashes, hives, eczema, vomiting, diarrhoea, and a rapid heart rate. Symptoms can appear immediately or within 24 hours, and can be mild or severe,

depending on how much of the allergen was consumed and the individual's sensitivity.

Some people suffer from an extreme reaction where their throat swells up so much that they have trouble breathing. This type of reaction to a food is rare, but life threatening.

Food allergies are most common in people with gastrointestinal disease and in infants. Once an infant's intestinal tract is fully developed, food allergies are less likely to occur. Many children who develop food allergies before three years of age will outgrow them, except for an allergy to peanuts. It's estimated that 5 per cent of infants and 1.5 per cent of young children suffer from a true food allergy, compared to 1 per cent of adults. Food allergies that appear after the age of three years are more likely to be a problem for life.

Although allergic reactions can occur to virtually any food, most reactions are caused by a small number of foods: eggs, cow's milk, nuts, soya beans, wheat, fish and seafood.

WHAT IS A FOOD INTOLERANCE?

Food intolerance (or food sensitivity) is the term used for adverse reactions to foods that are not caused by antibodies produced by the immune system. A food intolerance can be caused by chemicals or toxins that occur naturally in foods, or by substances added to foods during processing and preparation. Usually the more of the offending chemical that is eaten, the worse the symptoms.

Foods that are commonly thought to cause food intolerances include coffee, tea, red wine, beer, cocoa, chocolate, cow's milk, cheese, tomatoes, citrus fruit, processed meats, yeast and wheat. Unless it's obvious which foods cause your symptoms, you may need to use an elimination diet under the supervision of a doctor or dietitian to identify them.

FOOD ALLERGIES VERSUS FOOD INTOLERANCES

Excessive reactions to particular components in foods can be divided into two classes: food allergies and food intolerances.

Food allergies
- Food allergies are uncommon in adults, more common in children under five years of age and usually disappear with age.
- Reactions are more immediate and can be mild (rash, itchiness, watery eyes), severe or life threatening (throat closes and swells, breathing difficulties).
- Skin-prick tests can show which allergens you are sensitive to and blood tests can confirm the production of a specific antibody to the allergen.

Food intolerances
- Symptoms may develop over hours or even after days and are usually more vague (bloating, headache, flatulence, diarrhoea).
- Repeated exposure to the culprit chemical in foods may be necessary to reach a threshold level of the compound in the blood before a reaction occurs.

LACTOSE INTOLERANCE

People with lactose intolerance are unable to digest significant amounts of lactose, the main sugar in milk, because they don't produce enough of the enzyme lactase.

Lactase is normally produced in the gut of all humans at birth, so they can digest breast milk. Lactase levels tend to decrease with age and in many people decline so much that lactose can't be completely digested. In these people, any lactose they consume in dairy products will pass through the stomach into the large intestine, where it will be metabolised by bacteria. The undigested lactose, together with acids and gas produced by the bacteria, can result in flatulence, a bloated abdomen, cramping and diarrhoea.

The number of people with lactose intolerance varies in different ethnic groups, ranging from less than 5 per cent in Caucasians to almost 100 per cent of adults in some Asian and African societies that don't consume dairy products. People can also become lactose intolerant after an intestinal infection and other illnesses.

Because dairy products are a rich source of calcium, people with lactose intolerance must consume other sources of calcium to meet their needs. Some foods contain calcium with little or no lactose, such as sardines and salmon (eaten with bones), tofu processed in calcium salts, calcium-enriched soy milk and soy yoghurt, lactose-reduced milk, regular cheese and yoghurt. In most cases, small amounts of cow's milk can be tolerated.

GLUTEN INTOLERANCE (COELIAC DISEASE)

Coeliac disease is an illness in which the lining of the small intestine is damaged by gluten and similar proteins found in wheat, rye, oats, barley and triticale.

The disease tends to run in families, and can begin at any age, from infancy (after cereals have been introduced) until later in life (even if the person has been eating cereal grains for a long time), in response to some kind of physical or emotional stress.

Symptoms of coeliac disease vary depending on how much of the small intestine is affected. Gluten consumption can cause frequent diarrhoea resulting in dehydration and loss of minerals, which can lead to anaemia and osteoporosis. The reduced absorption of fat, carbohydrate and protein usually causes weight loss.

Coeliacs often suffer from other food sensitivities, particularly to lactose, alcohol, soy foods and MSG, which may also respond to a gluten-free diet.

FAT, FIBRE AND CARBOHYDRATE
Counter

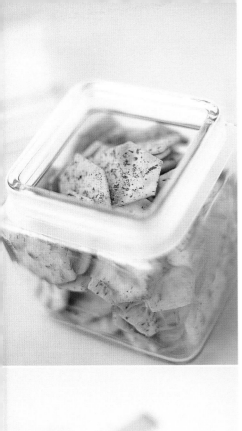

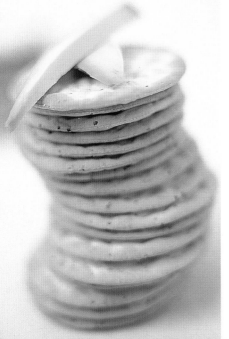

HOW TO USE THIS SECTION

Use the following few pages to identify your personal dietary needs, to understand the role of food in maintaining good health and to establish just how much nutrition your diet provides. The nutrition pages on labelling will then provide you with all the tools you need to identify what foods you should eat as part of a healthy diet.

The food composition chart shows the fibre, carbohydrate and energy values for most commonly available foods. The figure next to each food represents the average serving, but if the food has no typical serving, as is the case with flour, a 100g amount is given. In the fibre column, N denotes that the figure has not been calculated, + that amounts have been detected but not accurately calculated and Tr means that only a trace (less than 0.1g) has been found.

The right hand pages of the chart focus on particular foods, providing useful information about different varieties, healthy recipe variations, and hints and tips for making the foods part of a balanced diet. Essential tips on the best choices for everyday shopping are combined with notes on how to opt for lower-fat versions, and how taste needn't be compromised for health.

YOUR FAT & CARBOHYDRATE REQUIREMENTS

Everyone has different fat and carbohydrate requirements. The amount of calories you should be consuming each day depends on a number of different factors, including your age, sex, weight and activity level.

By following these four straightforward instructions, you can work out how many calories you need to consume every day in order to maintain a healthy and balanced diet. The results are only approximate – even those people who are the same sex, age, weight and activity level will have different energy requirements.

STEP I

The amount of calories you need each day depends both on your age and how much you weigh. In order to calculate your estimated calorie requirement, place your weight in kilograms in the appropriate equation for your age (see right).

STEP 2

Your body will require more or less calories depending on how active you are, both at work and during your leisure time. Multiply your calorie requirement from Step I by your activity level below. For example, if you are a woman and work in an office but do some form of exercise on most days, then your occupational activity level is 'light' but your non-occupational activity level will be 'moderately active'. So your overall activity level will be 1.5 (these levels are approximate).

STEP I – FOR MEN

18–29y	$[(0.063 \times weight) + 2.896] \times 239$
30–60y	$[(0.048 \times weight) + 3.653] \times 239$
Over 60y	$[(0.049 \times weight) + 2.459] \times 239$

STEP I – FOR WOMEN

18–29y	$[(0.062 \times weight) + 2.036] \times 239$
30–60y	$[(0.034 \times weight) + 3.538] \times 239$
Over 60y	$[(0.038 \times weight) + 2.755] \times 239$

Non-occupational activity	Occupational activity					
	light		moderate		moderate/heavy	
	male	female	male	female	male	female
Non-active	1.4	1.4	1.6	1.5	1.7	1.5
Moderately active	1.5	1.5	1.7	1.6	1.8	1.6
Very active	1.6	1.6	1.8	1.7	1.9	1.7

STEP 3

If you are trying to lose or gain weight, then you will need to reduce or increase the number of calories you consume every day. The best way of doing this is to subtract 500 calories from your estimated daily calorie needs. If you want to increase your weight, then add 500 calories. You have now calculated your average daily calorie needs.

The fact that you only need to reduce your calorie intake by 500 calories per day may come as a surprise to some people. However, this is by far the best way to go about dieting because it will enable you to lose 500g (1lb) per week. If you lose weight in a slow and steady manner, then you are much more likely to keep the weight off permanently than if you lose weight very quickly. Crash dieting is not the answer.

STEP 4

You can now calculate how many grams of fat and carbohydrate you should aim to eat each day for good health.

● No more than 35% of the calories you eat each day should come from fats. To calculate what this means in terms of the amount of fat you should be eating, place your calorie requirement into this equation:

$$\frac{(\text{calories/day} \times 0.35)}{9} = \text{grams fat each day}$$

● At least 50% of the calories you eat each day should come from carbohydrates. To calculate the grams of carbohydrates, place your calorie requirement into this equation:

$$\frac{(\text{calories} \times 0.5)}{3.75} = \text{grams carbohydrate each day}$$

SAMPLE CALCULATION

Jane is 36 years old, weighs 72kg and is 163cm tall. She has a 'light' occupation activity level and is moderately active out of work. She is trying to lose weight (see the Body Mass Index chart on page 17). Her estimated requirements are:

STEP 1 – Estimated calorie requirement

$[(0.034 \times 72) + 3.538] \times 239 = 1430$ calories / day

STEP 2 – Estimated calorie requirement determined by activity level

$1430 \times 1.5 = 2146$ calories / day

STEP 3 – Recommended calorie requirement to lose weight

$2146 - 500 = 1646$ calories / day

STEP 4 – Recommended fat and carbohydrate allowance per day

Grams of fat each day: $\dfrac{(1646 \times 0.35)}{9} = 64\text{g / day}$

Grams of carbohydrate each day: $\dfrac{(1646 \times 0.5)}{3.75} = 219\text{g / day}$

FINDING THE RIGHT BALANCE

Eating a wide variety of different foods in the right proportions and enjoying it is the key to a healthy diet! A combination of regular physical activity and a healthy diet not only helps you to stay in shape, but it also reduces your risk of developing conditions such as heart disease, cancer, constipation and osteoporosis.

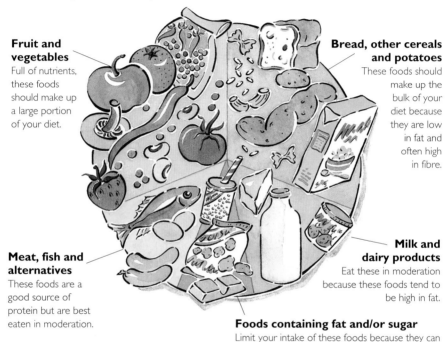

Fruit and vegetables
Full of nutrients, these foods should make up a large portion of your diet.

Bread, other cereals and potatoes
These foods should make up the bulk of your diet because they are low in fat and often high in fibre.

Meat, fish and alternatives
These foods are a good source of protein but are best eaten in moderation.

Milk and dairy products
Eat these in moderation because these foods tend to be high in fat.

Foods containing fat and/or sugar
Limit your intake of these foods because they can lead to obesity or tooth decay.

EATING A BALANCED DIET

There's no such thing as an 'unhealthy' food, only an 'unhealthy' diet. Therefore, eating healthily doesn't necessarily mean cutting out all your favourite foods but eating the right balance does mean eating more of some types of food than others. For example, at least half of the total calories that we eat should come from starchy foods, such as bread, potatoes, pasta and rice, which are high in carbohydrates. Fat should contribute

no more than 35% of the total calories that we eat. It can be difficult to know what this means in practical terms, but with the help of this book, eating healthily and maintaining a healthy weight will become second nature.

The diagram above, the food wheel, represents the recommended balance of foods in the diet, showing how much of each type of food we should aim to eat.

Bread, other cereals and potatoes

At least 50% of the calories we eat should come from the starchy foods included in this group. Because they are bulky, low in fat and often high in fibre, these foods fill us up without providing too many calories. It's what you serve with them (for example, butter on bread) that adds the fat and calories. This group also includes breakfast cereals, oats, pasta, noodles, plantains, beans and lentils. These foods provide carbohydrate (starch), some calcium and iron, and B vitamins. Make these foods the main part of most meals.

Fruit and vegetables

Eat plenty of these foods – aim for at least five portions a day (a glass of fruit juice can count as one portion). Choose from a wide variety of fresh, frozen or canned fruits and vegetables. Contrary to popular belief, frozen fruit and vegetables can be just as nutritious as fresh (if not more so) because they are usually frozen immediately after harvesting, reducing nutrient loss. They are full of antioxidant vitamins, especially vitamin C and carotenes (vitamin A), as well as folates, fibre and some carbohydrates. In addition, they are low in fat and calories.

Milk and dairy products

Eat moderate amounts of these foods and choose lower-fat alternatives where possible. This group includes milk, cheese, yoghurt and fromage frais, but it doesn't include butter, eggs and cream. Milk and dairy products provide calcium, protein, vitamins B12, A and D. Although semi-skimmed and skimmed milk contain less of the fat-soluble vitamins A and D, their calcium content is the same as full-fat milk.

Meat, fish and alternatives

Eat moderate amounts of these foods and choose lower-fat alternatives where possible. This group includes eggs, nuts, textured vegetable protein, tofu, beans and lentils. Aim to eat at least two portions of fish per week, one of which should be an oily fish. These foods provide iron, protein, B vitamins, zinc and magnesium.

Foods containing fat and/or sugar

Eat these types of foods sparingly and choose low-fat alternatives where possible. This group includes butter, other fat spreads, oils, salad dressings and treats such as biscuits, cakes, chocolate, ice cream, sweets, crisps and sweetened drinks. Sugary foods should be limited because eating them frequently can lead to tooth decay.

FATS

Small amounts of fat are essential to a healthy diet – they provide fat soluble vitamins A, D, E and K, as well as essential fatty acids.

Eating the right amount of fat

Most of us eat too much fat. Currently fat provides about 40% of the calories eaten. This needs to be reduced to no more than 35%. There are two main reasons why eating too much fat is bad for us:

- Fat contains more calories per gram (9kcal/g) than carbohydrates (3.75kcals/g), protein (4kcals/g) or alcohol (7kcals/g). This means that foods containing a high proportion of fat tend to be high in calories. So, eating them in large amounts is likely to lead to weight gain and obesity.

- Eating too much fat, especially saturated fat, increases the risk that you might develop heart disease.

Eating the right sort of fat

It's not just the total amount of fat we eat that can affect our health, but also the type of fat. Fat is made up of units called fatty acids and there are three main types of fatty acids – saturated, monounsaturated and polyunsaturated. The fat in food contains a mixture of all three types, but different foods contain different proportions of each type.

Saturated fat

Foods that contain a high proportion of saturated fats include some milk and dairy products and meat and meat products. They are also found in palm and coconut oil and some spreading fats, hard cooking fats, biscuits, cakes and pastries. Eating too much saturated fat increases levels of blood cholesterol. Cholesterol is made mostly by the liver and is carried in the blood by proteins called LDL's and HDL's. LDL cholesterol is sometimes referred to as 'bad' cholesterol because high blood levels can result in cholesterol being deposited on the blood vessel walls, eventually leading to atherosclerosis and possibly a heart attack. HDL cholesterol, on the other hand, is often referred to as 'good' cholesterol because it carries the cholesterol to the liver for disposal.

Monounsaturated fats

Monounsaturates are the main type of fat found in olive and rapeseed oils. They are also found in some spreading fats, nuts, avocados, milk and dairy products and meat. When saturates in the diet are replaced by monounsaturated, 'bad' cholesterol levels are reduced and the risk of heart disease lowered.

Polyunsaturated fats

There are two main groups of polyunsaturates known as n-6 and n-3 according to their structure. When saturates in the diet are replaced by n-6 polyunsaturates (found in sunflower, corn and soya bean oils, spreads high in polyunsaturates and meat), levels of 'bad' cholesterol in the blood are reduced. However, it is likely that 'good' cholesterol levels are also reduced. Current dietary guidelines recommend that we do not increase our intake of polyunsaturates any further and that we should aim to replace the saturates in our diet with monoun-saturates as well as polyunsaturates.

n-3 polyunsaturates are the main types of fat found in oily fish such as mackerel, pilchards, sardines, trout and salmon. These fats are sometimes referred to as omega-3 fatty acids and some spreading fats are now enriched with them. These types of fats have no effect on blood cholesterol levels, but they do reduce the tendency of blood to clot, thereby reducing the risk of heart disease.

Trans fatty acids

Trans fatty acids (trans fats) occur naturally in dairy foods such as butter, and fat from beef and lamb. They are also produced during margarine manufacture. This process, hydrogenation, produces hydrogenated fats. If hydrogenated fats/oils are included in an ingredients list, this indicates that a food contains trans fats. This fat is often found in spreading fats, biscuits and cakes. Trans fats may have undesirable effects on cholesterol levels (in a similar way to saturated fats) and you should limit the amount you eat.

What about cholesterol intake?

Did you know that the amount of cholesterol we eat has only a very small effect on the amount of cholesterol in our blood? If we eat large quantities of cholesterol, the body responds by producing less, so the overall effect on blood cholesterol levels will be small. Increasing saturated fat intake and becoming obese are the most likely causes of increasing blood cholesterol levels.

FIBRE

Fibre is the non-digestible part of food. It includes two types of fibre: soluble and insoluble. The soluble fibre, which is found in oats, pulses, fruit and vegetables, may help lower blood cholesterol levels if consumed as part of a diet low in saturated fats. The insoluble fibre found in foods such as bread, pasta, rice and cereals reduces constipation and the risk of other bowel disorders.

On average, we eat about 12g of fibre a day. According to healthy eating guidelines, this should be increased to 18g per day. The two food groups 'bread, other cereals and potatoes' and 'fruit and vegetables' illustrated in the food wheel on page 14 are good sources of dietary fibre. Making sure that these foods make up two-thirds of your diet would significantly increase your fibre intake.

Are you a healthy weight?

Health experts use Body Mass Index (BMI) to assess people's weight. You can calculate your own BMI by using the following equation or by simply plotting your weight on the chart below:

weight (kg)/ height² (m) = BMI
eg 72kg/1.63²m = 27 BMI

BMI criteria	
Less than 18	Underweight
18–20	OK – a healthy weight but do not lose any more
20–25	OK – a healthy weight
25–30	Overweight
30–40	Fat
Over 40	Very fat

Body Mass Index Chart

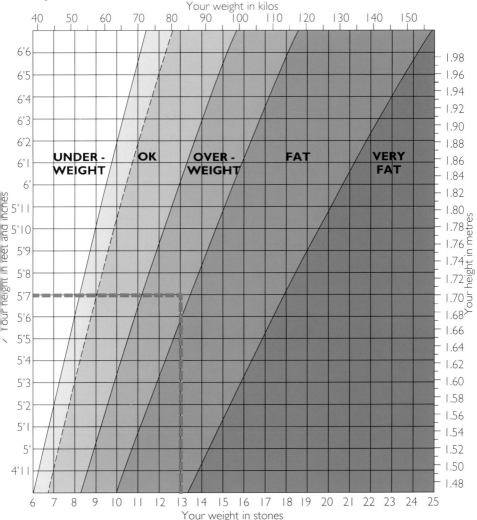

NUTRITION LABELLING

Reading nutrition labels can tell you a lot about the food you are eating, which is important if you want to eat a healthy, balanced diet. But understanding the information can be tricky, so here's a brief guide to help you.

Food packets contain a great deal of information about the food inside but they can sometimes be confusing or even misleading. You can often learn something about the food from its name. Certain foods are required by law to be sold under prescribed names, such as margarine, ice cream and bread, which contain specified quantities of ingredients. The manufacturer is also required to state a contact name and address, and list the food's country of origin, which can either mean the country in which the food was grown or in which it was packaged.

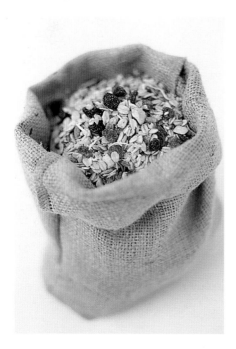

What a nutrition label tells you

Regulations differ from country to country but most governments require that any packaged foods displaying a nutritional claim (for example, 'low fat'), must also display nutrition labelling. If no claim is made on the packaging then manufacturers do not have to show nutrition information. Nutrition labels have to show the amount of energy, protein, carbohydrate and fat in 100g of the food. Values for sugar, saturated fat, fibre and sodium are also sometimes given. Labels making specific claims have to show values for the nutrient about which the claim is made.

Nutrition Information

Typical Values	Per fipizza	Per 100g (3.5oz)
Energy	2316kJ	1158kJ
	550kcals	275kcals
Protein	25.0g	12.5g
Carbohydrate	70.8g	35.4g
of which sugars	5.2g	2.6g
of which starch	65.6g	32.8g
Fat	18.6g	9.3g
of which saturates	6.8g	3.4g
Monounsaturates	6.4g	3.2g
Polyunsaturates	4.6g	2.3g
Fibre	3.4g	1.7g
Sodium	1.4g	0.7g

* For definitions of the above nutrients see Food Terms on pages 218–223.

Ingredients list

Ingredients are listed by weight – the one present in the largest amount appears first and others are listed in descending order (except water). You can use ingredients lists to compare products for value or to help you avoid ingredients you don't want to eat.

Per serving or per 100g

Although it's often more useful to have nutrition values 'per serving' of food, manufacturers have to give values per 100g as well. This is useful for comparing the nutrient content of two different foods. You can still calculate the nutrient content of a portion by dividing the amounts in 100g by the weight of your portion (g)/100.

The weight of the food in a package is normally given on the label accompanied by a big ℮ (for example, 250ml ℮). This means that the average quantity of food must be accurate, but that the weight of each packet may vary slightly.

Nutrition claims

In most countries there are guidelines that most food manufacturers and retailers use to govern the meaning of some nutrition claims. However, not all claims are covered by these guidelines and not all food manufacturers stick to them when they are. Claims can also be quite misleading. For example if a product says 'reduced fat' this means that it should contain at least 25% less fat than the standard product, but in the case of biscuits or crisps, for example the product is likely still to be relatively high in fat. The only way to be sure is to read the nutrition label. Here's what some of the common claims should mean:

Claim	Meaning
'low fat' or 'low sugar'	No more than 5g of fat or sugar per 100g food.
'low saturates'	No more than 3g saturated fat per 100g food.
'reduced fat' or 'reduced sugar'	The product must contain at least 25% less fat or sugar than the standard product.
'low sodium'	No more than 40mg per 100g.

'high fibre'	More than 6g per 100g.
'fat free' 'saturates free'	No more than 0.15g per 100g. No more than 0.1g per 100g.
'sugar free'	No more than 0.2g per 100g.
'no added sugar'	No sugars or foods composed mainly of sugars (for example, dried fruit or concentrated fruit juice) should be added to the food or any of its ingredients.

The following claims are not covered by voluntary government guidelines and may mean something different each time, the only way to be really sure is by checking the label:

Light or Lite: this could mean light in weight, light in colour or more often low in fat.

Half fat: this means that the food contains half the fat of its standard counterpart.

Lower fat: this usually means that the food contains less fat than its standard counterpart, but how much lower can only be ascertained by reading the labels. The chances are, it's not that much lower otherwise it would be covered by the 'low fat' or 'reduced fat' claim.

Virtually fat free: this usually means there is very little fat in a food. But remember, if a label says '90% fat free' it also means it contains 10% fat, which means that the product can't be classified as low fat!

'Diet' products

According to food labelling regulations the word 'diet' can only appear on products that make a 'low calorie' claim. To classify as a low calorie food, a food must contain no more than 40 calories per 100g or 100ml (in the case of drinks) or per serving if less than 100g. The claim must also be accompanied by the statement '...can help slimming or weight control only as part of a calorie controlled diet.'

FOOD	CARB g	FIBRE g	FAT g	ENERGY kcal	kJ
ALCOHOL					
Beers					
ale, brown, bottled – small, 275ml	8.3	0	0	82	346
ale, pale, bottled – small, 275ml	5.5	0	0	77	325
ale, strong – small, 275ml	17	0	0	182	756
beer, average, 1 pint, 574ml	13	0	0	182	756
beer, bitter, canned, 440ml	10.3	0	0	143	586
beer, bitter, canned, large, 500ml	11.6	0	0	161	660
beer, bitter, low alcohol, 1 pint, 574ml	12	0	0	75	310
beer, draught, 1 pint, 574ml	13.3	0	0	184	755
beer, keg, 1 pint, 574ml	13.2	0	0	178	741
beer, mild, draught, 1 pint, 574ml	9.3	0	0	145	597
lager, average, canned and draught, 500ml	Tr	0	0	145	605
lager, bottled, large, 500ml	7.5	0	0	146	598
lager, reduced-alcohol, 1 pint, 574ml	8.6	0	0	57.4	235
lager, premium, strong, 500ml	Tr	0	0	295	1220
shandy, canned, large, 500ml	15	0	0	55	240
stout, bottled, small, 275ml	11.4	0	0	100	429
stout, strong, large, 500ml	10.5	0	0	195	817
stout, strong, small, 275ml	5.8	0	0	107	449
Ciders					
cider, dry, 1 pint, 574ml	15	0	0	208	873
cider, sweet, 1 pint, 574ml	24.4	0	0	244	1011
cider, vintage, strong, 1 pint, 574ml	42	0	0	578	2417
Cocktails					
cocktail, Bloody Mary, 165ml	5.5	0.5	0	124	520
cocktail, Daiquiri, 60ml	4	0	0	111	465
cocktail, Tequila Sunrise, 60ml	7	0	0	66	275
Liqueurs					
liqueur, egg-based, 25ml	7	0	1.6	65	273
liqueur, cherry brandy/coffee, 25ml	8.2	0	0	65.5	275
liqueur, cream, 25ml	6	0	4	81	338
liqueur, drambuie, 25ml	6.1	0	0	78.5	330
Spirits					
spirits, average, 40% volume – brandy, gin, rum, vodka, whiskey, 25ml	0	0	0	55	230
spirits, average, 37.5% volume, 25ml	0	0	0	51	214
Wines					
wine, red, small glass, 120ml	0.4	0	0	85	356
wine, rose, 120ml	3.1	0	0	89	367
wine, white, dry, 120ml	0.7	0	0	82	343
wine, white, medium, 120ml	4.3	0	0	94	388
wine, white, sweet, 120ml	7.4	0	0	118	493
wine, fortified, port, 50ml	6	0	0	80	327
wine, fortified, sherry, dry, 50ml	0.7	0	0	58	240
wine, fortified, sherry, medium, 50ml	3	0	0	60	252
wine, fortified, sherry, sweet, 50ml	3.5	0	0	68	284
wine, fortified, vermouth, dry, 50ml	1.5	0	0	55	227

ALCOHOL Drinking alcohol in moderate amounts (no more than 2 to 3 units a day for women, or 3 to 4 units for men), does not appear to have any adverse health effects in adults of a healthy weight. However, do have at least one or two alcohol-free days a week and avoid binge drinking. Try to limit alcohol to meal times.

BEER A drink made by the fermentation of cereals (usually barley), beer can be high in calories and may also weaken resolve when it comes to reaching for high-fat snacks.

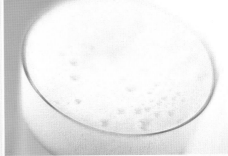

RECIPE For a refreshing summer drink with just 65 calories, pour about 60ml of dry sparkling wine and 60ml of soda water over berries and allow to stand for a few minutes.

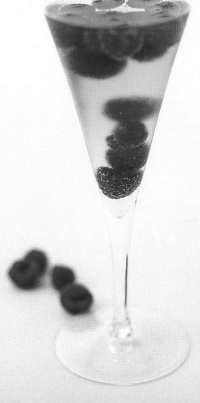

WHITE WINE Mix with ice-cold soda water to make a wine spritzer with half the calories of a glass of wine.

SPIRITS Adding full-sugar mixers or juice to a spirit increases the calorie content. Try diet mixers or soda water for a change.

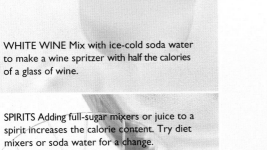

FOOD	CARB g	FIBRE g	FAT g	ENERGY kcal	ENERGY kJ
ALCOHOL CONT.					
wine, fortified, vermouth, sweet, 50ml	7.6	0	0	75	315
champagne, 125ml	1.7	0	0	95	394
APPLE					
chutney, 1 serving, 35g	18	0.6	0	68	288
cooking, stewed with sugar, 4oz, 100g	19	1.8	0	74	314
cooking, stewed without sugar, 4oz, 100g	8	2	0	33	138
eating, raw, unpeeled, 1 average, 5oz, 125g	13	2.2	0	52.5	224
eating, raw, peeled, 1 average, 4oz, 100g	11	0	0	45	190
dried, 1oz, 25g	15	2.4	0	60	254
juice, unsweetened, small glass, 4fl oz, 100ml	10	Tr	0	38	164
juice, concentrated, 1fl oz, 25g	14	Tr	0	57	243
APRICOT					
canned in juice, 6 halves, 120g	9.6	1.2	0	41	176
canned in syrup, 6 halves, 120g	19	1.2	0	76	321
raw, 3, 110g	6.8	2	0	28	119
stewed with sugar, 4oz serving, 100g	18	2	0	72	308
stewed without sugar, 4oz serving, 100g	6	2	0	27	115
dried, 3 whole, 50g	22	4	0	94	401
ready to eat – semi-dried, 4oz, 100g	36	6.3	0	158	674
juice drink, 35% juice, 1 glass, 250ml	20	1	0	18	75
nectar, 50% juice, glass, 250ml	32	0	0	129	540
ARTICHOKE					
globe, boiled, 1 medium, 220g	2.6	1	0	17	70
hearts, canned in brine, drained, 1 heart, 50g	1	1.5	0	8	35
Jerusalem, peeled, boiled, 1 medium, 100g	10	3.5	0	41	207
ASPARAGUS					
canned, drained, 8 spears, 100g	1.5	2.9	0	24	100
fresh, boiled, 4 spears, 120g	1	1	0	15	63
AUBERGINE (see also EGGPLANT)					
fried in corn oil, 100g	2.8	2.3	32	302	1262
raw, 100g	2.2	2	0.4	15	64
AVOCADO					
medium, 1 raw 100g	1.9	3.4	19.5	190	784
BABY FOOD					
baby rusk, plain, average, 100g	82.8	N	7.9	408	1729
rusk, flavoured, 100g	78.1	N	9	401	1698
rusk, low sugar, 100g	77.8	N	9.7	414	1751
rusk, wholemeal, 100g	76.5	N	10.1	411	1739
cereal, ground muesli, 100g	70	N	8	400	1690
cereal, creamed porridge, 100g	58	N	5.5	360	1510
cereal, mixed, powder, 100g	71	N	5	377	1599
cereal, fruit, banana & apple, powder, 100g	70	N	3.8	359	1527
cereal, apple & blackberry, powder, 100g	77	N	4	365	1552
baby rice, powder, 100g	78	N	3	365	1553
baby rice, mixed, 100g	78	N	2	372	1565
dessert, creamed rice, jar, 128g	8	0	0.5	40	155
dessert, fruit, powder, 100g	90	1.3	0.6	383	1635

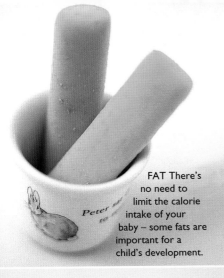

FAT There's no need to limit the calorie intake of your baby – some fats are important for a child's development.

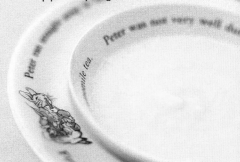

BEST FOR BABY Breast or formula milk is the only food that babies need for the first 4–6 months. Breast milk is particularly ideal because it provides all the necessary nutrients, together with certain antibodies that help protect young babies from infection.

BABY FOOD Most babies are

ready for 'solid' foods by about the age of 4 months. Keep things simple to start with, by offering puréed fruit or vegetables, with no added salt or sugar. Try to keep commercially produced baby foods to a minimum, and always check labels to ensure that the food is suitable for your child.

FIBRE Babies only have small stomachs and need to obtain a lot of nutrients from small portions. Foods high in fibre such as wholewheat cereals and/or wholemeal bread can be filling, without providing sufficient energy, so avoid offering them every day.

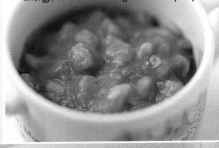

RECIPE To make a nutritious and tasty 'first food' for your baby, steam some swede (or pumpkin) and potato until tender. Purée and add a little breast or formula milk and then pass through a sieve in order to remove any lumps.

FOOD	CARB	FIBRE	FAT	ENERGY	
	g	g	g	kcal	kJ
BABY FOOD CONT.					
dessert, caramel custard, 100g	13	N	2.5	82	345
dessert, fruit custard, 100g	17	N	0.5	74	310
dinner, beef, junior, 100g	10	1	0.5	60	240
dinner, chicken & vegetable, 100g	8	1.5	1.5	60	250
dinner, chicken, junior, 100g	9	0.5	1	55	230
dinner, chicken noodle, junior, 100g	9.5	0.5	1	57	240
egg/cheese based meal, canned, 100g	10	1	3.4	82	344
meat based meal, average, canned, 100g	8.6	1.1	3	73	306
dinner, lamb casserole, jar 200g	18	N	2	121	510
dinner, lamb, junior, 100g	7	1	2.5	62	260
dinner, lentil hot-pot, jar, 200g	20	N	0.5	114	480
dinner, fish based, average, canned, 100g	9	0.6	3	76	321
dinner, garden vegetable, jar, 200g	24	N	0.5	124	520
dinner, mixed vegetable, strained, 100g	8.5	N	1	46	195
dinner, pasta & vegetable, jar, 200g	27	N	1	138	580
dinner, pasta based, average, canned, 100g	8.5	0.7	3	71	300
dinner, vegetable based, canned, 100g	10	2	2	67	284
BACON					
bits, 2tsp	0	0	1.5	30	125
fried & 2 fried eggs	0	0	18	215	905
middle rasher, fried, 1 slice, 10g	0	0	3	37	155
middle rasher, trimmed, fried, 1, 10g	0	0	1	23	95
middle rasher, grilled, 1, 10g	0	0	2	32	135
middle rasher, trimmed, grilled, 1, 10g	0	0	1	24	100
BAGEL					
plain, average, 1, 60g	29	+	0.5	137	575
BAKLAVA					
bought, average piece, 100g	40	+	17.5	322	1349
BAMBOO SHOOTS					
canned or bottled, drained, 1 cup, 140g	1.5	2.2	0	11	45
raw, 50g	3	N	0	14.3	60
BANANA					
chips, crystallised, 1oz, approx. 25 chips, 25g	15	0.5	7.8	128	534
dried, 100g	28	3	0	119	500
raw, peeled, 140g	32.5	1	Tr	133	564
BARLEY					
bran, raw, 40g	30	+	1	131	550
cooked, 1 portion, 180g	38	+	1.5	190	800
pearl, cooked, 100g	27.7	+	1	120	510
wholegrain, raw, 100g	64	15	2	301	1282
BEANS AND LENTILS					
aduki, cooked, 4oz portion, 100g	22.5	5.5	0.2	123	525
baked, canned in tomato sauce, 100g	15	3.5	0.6	81	345
balor, canned in salted water, 100g	2.8	2.7	0.1	19	83
black-eyed, cooked, 100g	20	3.5	0.7	116	494
black gram, cooked, 100g	13.5	N	0.4	89	379
black kidney, cooked, 100g	24.5	N	0.5	130	545

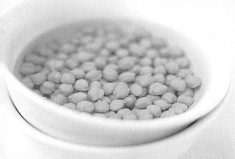

KIDNEY BEANS Next time you make chilli con carne, try using more kidney beans and less beef mince, as kidney beans are high in fibre and supply all the protein of meat without the fat.

CHICKPEAS Readily available in tins, chickpeas are a great source of fibre and a cheap, low-fat alternative to meat.

BEANS Rich in protein, dietary fibre and complex carbohydrates, and low in fat, beans should be an essential part of our diet, especially for people who don't eat any or much meat. The canned varieties are great if you don't have time to soak dried beans overnight.

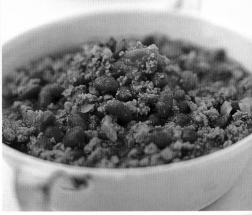

SOYA BEANS An excellent source of phytoestrogens (compounds which may have some beneficial effects in menopausal women), soya beans also provide the best quality protein of all the pulses.

RECIPE Process chickpeas with a little tahini, garlic, lemon juice, oil and water to make a delicious low-fat dip. Serve with pieces of wholemeal bread or warmed pitta bread.

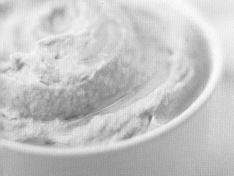

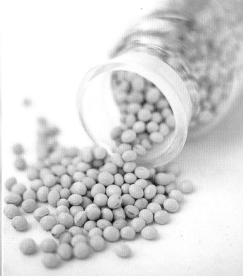

FOOD	CARB.	FIBRE	FAT	ENERGY	
	g	g	g	kcal	kJ

BEANS AND LENTILS CONT.

FOOD	CARB.	FIBRE	FAT	kcal	kJ
borlotti, canned, drained, 100g	25	N	0.5	112	470
borlotti, cooked, 100g	28.5	N	0.5	146	612
broad, fresh, cooked, 100g	5.6	5.4	0.8	48	204
butter (cannellini), canned, 100g	13	4.6	0.5	77	327
chickpeas, canned, drained, 100g portion	16	4.1	2.9	115	487
green, fresh, cooked, 100g	3	2.4	0	22	92
green, frozen, cooked, 100g	4.7	4.1	0	25	108
haricot, cooked, 100g	17.2	6.1	0.5	95	406
kidney, red, canned, drained, cooked, 100g	12.2	4.1	0.5	70	380
lentils, canned in tomato sauce, 100g	9.3	1.7	0.2	55	236
lentils, red, split, cooked, 100g	17.5	2	0.4	100	424
lentils, whole, dried, cooked, 100g	17	3.8	0.7	105	446
lima, dried, cooked, 100g	10	5.5	Tr	70	295
mung, cooked, 100g	15.3	10	0.4	91	389
pinto, cooked, 100g	24	N	0.7	137	583
red kidney bean, cooked, 100g	17.4	6.7	0.5	103	440
red kidney beans, in chilli sauce,100g	13.1	3.6	2.6	91	383
runner, fresh, cooked, 100g	2.3	1.9	0.5	18	76
soya, canned, drained, 100g	5.1	6.1	7.3	141	590
soya, canned in tomato sauce, 100g	7	3	3	90	380
soya, dried, cooked, 100g	1.5	6.1	7.5	128	540
three-bean mix, canned, drained, 100g	14	N	0.5	86	360
tofu, soya bean, steamed, 100g	0.7	N	4.2	73	304

BEEF

FOOD	CARB.	FIBRE	FAT	kcal	kJ
steak, lean, grilled, 1 medium, 117g	0	0	10.5	224	940
steak, untrimmed, grilled, 1, 120g	0	0	12.5	250	1040
chuck steak, untrimmed, simmered, 1, 190g	0	0	26	486	2040
corned, canned, 100g	0	0	12.5	217	905
corned, sliced, 100g	0	0	9	150	625
fillet steak, lean, grilled, 1, small, 85g	0	0	7	167	700
fillet steak, untrimmed, grilled, 1 small, 85g	0	0	11	198	830
Beef burgers, grilled, 100g	0.1	0	24.4	326	1355
homemade, 100g	1	0	20	287	1194
takeaway, in bun with salad, 100g	18	N	12.7	238	996
economy, frozen, grilled, 100g	9.7	0.8	19.3	273	1138
heart, simmered, 100g	0	0	5.9	179	752
kidney, simmered, 100g	0	0	6.1	153	641
liver, simmered, 100g	0	0	9.5	198	831
mince, simmered, drained, 170g	0	0	20.5	390	1623
mince, lean, simmered, drained, 170g	0	0	16.5	309	1300
oxtail, simmered, 100g	0	0	13.5	243	1014
pepper steak with cream sauce, 1 serving, 200g	0	0	35	536	2250
pie, bought, family size, 1 serving, 250g	38.5	+	36.5	560	2355
pie, bought, individual, 250g	45	+	34.5	564	2370
pie, bought, party size, 1, 40g	7.5	+	7.5	111	465
rib steak, lean, grilled, 100g	0	0	5.5	176	740
rissoles, fried, 2, 340g	0	+	30	662	2780

CASSEROLES To make your casseroles lower in calories but still full of flavour, prepare one day in advance and refrigerate overnight. Before reheating, carefully lift off and discard the fat that will have risen and set on the surface.

MINCE To make really lean mince, buy lean steak and mince it yourself in a food processor. Alternatively, buy extra lean mince, cook without fat and drain off all juices.

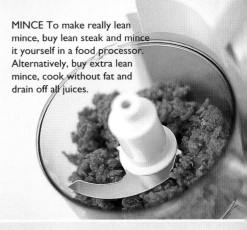

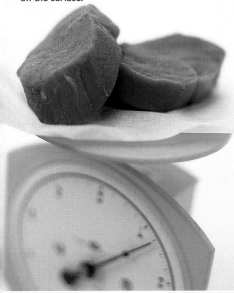

BEEF Lean beef, cooked without any added fat, can contain as little as 5% fat. Moderate amounts of red meat, such as beef, can be part of a healthy balanced diet and is an excellent source of iron and other minerals. Choose lean cuts that have had all visible fat removed and use low-fat marinades, such as lemon juice, mustard, soy sauce and herbs.

RECIPE To give a fillet steak extra flavour when you are grilling or frying it without fat, baste with a little marinade of soy sauce, spread both sides with wholegrain mustard or coat in cracked black pepper.

COOKING To avoid adding extra fat, cook your meat on a lightly oiled griddle pan or barbecue, but don't turn the meat too often and allow to rest before serving to keep it from drying out.

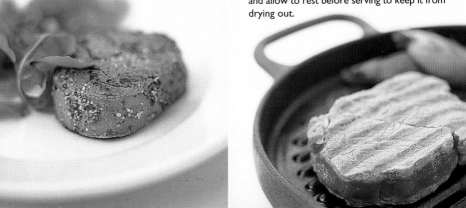

FOOD	CARB g	FIBRE g	FAT g	ENERGY kcal	kJ
BEEF CONT.					
round steak, lean, grilled, 100g	0	0	6	176	740
round steak, untrimmed, grilled, 100g	0	0	9.5	202	850
rump steak, lean, grilled, 175g	0	0	11.5	334	1405
rump steak, untrimmed, grilled, 200g	0	0	33.5	538	2260
silverside, lean, baked, 2 slices, 80g	0	0	3.5	131	550
silverside, untrimmed, baked, 2 slices, 85g	0	0	10	189	795
sirloin steak, lean, grilled, 110g	0	0	9.5	192	806
sirloin steak, untrimmed, grilled, 127g	0	0	24	348	1460
skirt steak, lean, simmered, 100g	0	0	5	188	790
skirt steak, untrimmed, simmered, 100g	0	0	6	196	825
steak, lean, grilled, 1 small, 110g	0	0	9	216	910
steak, untrimmed, grilled, 1 small, 130g	0	0	20.5	330	1390
T-bone, lean, grilled, 100g	0	0	5.5	134	565
T-bone, untrimmed, grilled, 100g	0	0	8	164	690
tongue, simmered, 100g	0	0	25	307	1290
topside roast, lean, baked, 2 slices. 80g	0	0	4	124	520
topside roast, untrimmed, baked, 2 slices, 90g	0	0	9	171	720
topside steak, lean, grilled,1 small, 100g	0	0	5	151	635
topside steak, untrimmed, grilled, 1 small,100g	0	0	6.5	162	680
tripe, simmered, 100g	0	0	3	83	350
BEETROOT					
fresh, peeled, boiled, 2 slices	5	0.4	0	25	105
pickled, 5 slices, 100g	14	1.7	0	64	270
raw, grated, 30g	2.5	0.6	0	12	50
BISCUITS					
assorted creams, 1, 15g	12.5	N	4	75	315
brandy snaps, 1, 10g	6.4	Tr	2	44	183
bourbon, 1, 12.5g	8.5	N	3.2	64	270
chocolate, full coated, 1 small, 25g	17	0.6	7	131	549
chocolate coated, 2, 30g	20	0.9	7.2	148	621
chocolate chip cookies, 1	4.5	N	2	36	150
chocolate shortbreads, 1	5	N	2.5	35	147
choc-chip, 1, 10g	8	N	2	51	215
cookies, 1, 10g	9	N	2.5	62	260
coconut ice, 1	9.5	+	3.5	71	300
cream biscuit, 1, 10g	6.4	N	2	46	194
custard cream, 1, 12.5g	8	N	3	64	270
digestive biscuits, plain, 2, 30g	20	0.7	6.3	141	593
digestive biscuit, chocolate, 1, 15g	10	0.3	3.6	74	311
flapjacks, 1, 25g	15	0.7	6.5	121	552
ginger nuts, 2, 20g	16	0.4	3	91	385
gingernut biscuits, homemade, 1, 20g	13	0.3	3.4	90	377
golden oat, 1, 15g	9.5	0.5	1.5	54	225
jaffa cake, 2	7	N	1	36	153
melting moments, 1, 10g	5.5	0.1	3.6	55	229
oatcakes, homemade, 1, 10g	6.3	0.6	1.8	44.5	187
oatcakes, retail, 1, 10g	6.3	N	1.8	44	185

BISCUITS Sweet biscuits are often high in sugar and saturated fat, but they can be useful as a quick source of carbohydrate. If you want something lower in fat to snack on, reach for fresh or dried fruit, or a crispbread or rice cake with cottage cheese. Alternatively, baking your own biscuits will help you cut back on fat and sugar.

SHORTBREAD High in fat and sugar, that lovely melt-in-the-mouth texture comes from the high ratio of butter to flour.

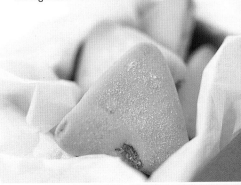

COOKIES Chewy ones get their texture from the high amount of butter and sugar. Don't be fooled into thinking oatmeal biscuits are lower in fat, though they do contain more fibre.

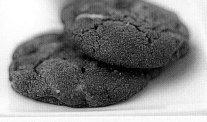

BISCOTTI A great low-fat biscuit. Made with eggs, they contain no butter and they also have extra fibre because they contain nuts.

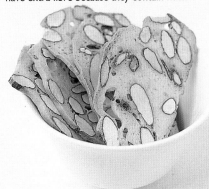

CREAM-FILLED High in fat and sugar, the centre is usually a mix of icing sugar, butter and water, and in most cases the biscuit is sweet and buttery.

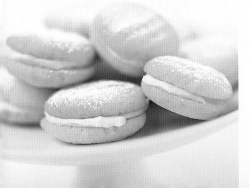

LOW-FAT There are biscuits now available in supermarkets that are up to 70% lower in fat than normal biscuits but they are still relatively high in fat and sugar.

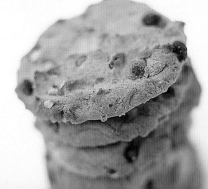

FOOD	CARB	FIBRE	FAT	ENERGY	
	g	g	g	kcal	kJ
BISCUITS CONT.					
fruit slice, 1, 15g	8	+	0.5	37	155
sandwich biscuit, 2, 25g	17.3	N	6.5	128	538
semi-sweet, 2, 15g	11.2	0.3	2.5	69	289
semi-sweet, coconut type, 1, 10g	9	0.1	2	56	23
semi-sweet, morning coffee type, 1, 12g	4.5	0.1	1	30	126
semi-sweet, rich tea type, 1, 7.5g	5.6	0.1	1.2	35	145
short-sweet biscuit, 2, 20g	12.4	0.3	4.7	94	393
shortbread, 2 fingers, 35g	22	0.8	9	174	730
shortbread, cream, 1	10.5	0	4.5	87	365
shortbread, scotch finger, 1	12	0.5	4	88	370
shortcake, 2, 20g	12	0.3	5	94	393
wafers, filled, 3, 18g	12	N	5.4	96	404
savoury, biscuit, 1	2	N	0.5	14	60
savoury, crackers, cream, 3, 21g	14.3	0.6	3.4	92	390
savoury, crackers, wholemeal, 3, 21g	15	1	2.4	87	366
crispbread, cracotte type, 3, 15g	9.4	0.4	2.3	61	256
crispbread, rye, 3, 24g	17	2.8	0.5	77	328
matzos, 1, 30g	26	1	0.6	115	490
oatcakes, 2, 26g	16.4	1.2	4.8	115	482
water biscuits, 3, 21g	16	0.6	2.6	92	390
BLACKBERRIES					
canned, sweetened, 100g	23	+	0	92	385
fresh, raw, ½ punnet, 100g	12.5	3.1	0.5	52	220
frozen, 100g	15.5	+	0.5	64	270
BLACKCURRANT JUICE					
prepared, diluted, 250ml	28	0	0	107	450
BLUEBERRIES					
canned in syrup, drained, 100g	17	+	0	69	290
frozen, 100g	12	+	0.5	51	215
raw, ½ punnet, 100g	14	1.8	0.5	56	235
BOYSENBERRIES					
canned in heavy syrup, 100g	22.5	2.6	0	88	370
canned, no added sugar, 100g	4	+	0	27	115
raw, ½ punnet, 100g	6	+	0	13	55
BRAN (see CEREAL)					
BRANDY BUTTER					
1tbsp, 30g	16	0	8	146	615
BRAWN					
2 slices, 70g	0	0	12	151	635
BREAD					
bagel, plain, average, 1, 60g	29	+	0.5	137	575
breadcrumbs, homemade, 100g	77.5	2.2	1.9	354	1508
breadcrumbs, manufactured, 100g	78.5	N	2.1	354	1505
brown bread, average, 38g	16.8	1.3	0.8	83	352
brown roll, crusty, 48g	24.2	1.7	1.3	122	521
brown roll, soft, 48g	24.9	1.7	1.8	129	547
chapatis, made with fat, 1, 100g	48.3	N	12.8	328	1383

FLAVOURED CRACKERS These can be high in fat and salt, so always check the nutrition label for full information.

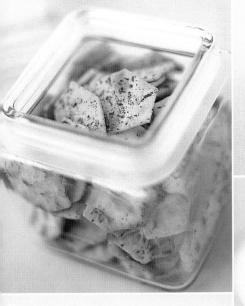

BISCUITS, CRACKERS & CRISPBREADS

Some savoury biscuits, such as rice crackers and oatcakes, are low in fat and sugar, and make a good alternative to bread. However, be aware that some savoury biscuits can be high in fat and salt. Choose wholewheat or high fibre varieties to boost your fibre intake.

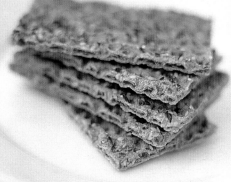

WATER CRACKERS Relatively fat-free, these crackers are a good source of carbohydrate. Serve them with low-fat soft cheese or yogurt dips, salad vegetables or reduced fat hummus.

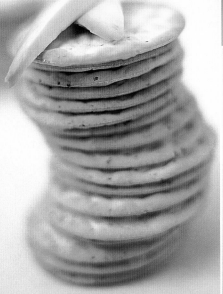

CRISPBREADS A high-fibre choice for an afternoon snack. Top with some cottage or low-fat soft cheese and slices of ripe tomato.

RICE CRACKERS A tasty low-fat cracker that provides a handy gluten-free snack high in carbohydrate.

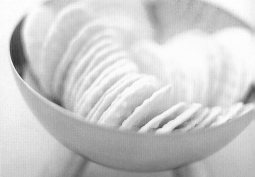

FOOD	CARB g	FIBRE g	FAT g	ENERGY kcal	kJ
BREAD CONT.					
chapatis, made without fat, 1, 100g	43.7	N	1	202	860
corn, 90g	20	+	7	178	750
croissant, 60g	23	1	12.2	216	903
crumpet, wholemeal, toasted, 1, 44g	17	1.5	0.5	84	355
currant bread, 1 slice, 25g	12.7	+	1.9	72	305
focaccia, 1, 50g	30	2	1.5	139	585
focaccia, herb & garlic, 1, 70g	32	2	1.5	170	715
granary, 1 slice, 38g	17.6	1.6	1	89	380
hamburger roll, 85g	41.5	1.3	4.3	224	953
loaf, average, white, 2 slices	35	3.5	2	189	795
loaf, fruit, fruit & spice, 2 slices	34.5	+	2	177	745
loaf, fruit, raisin toast, 2 slices	26	+	1.5	134	565
loaf, fruit, spicy fruit, 2 slices	33.5	+	2	174	730
loaf, gluten/wheat free, 2 slices	12	+	2	64	270
loaf, mixed grain, 2 slices	33.5	+	3.5	196	825
loaf, multi-grains, 2 slices	35	+	2	187	785
loaf, pumpernickel, 2 slices	18	3.7	1	92	385
loaf, rice bran, 2 slices	2	+	10	69	290
loaf, black rye, 1 slice	42	+	2	214	900
loaf, rye, 2 slices	30	2.2	3	176	740
loaf, soya & linseed, 2 slices	40	++	6	259	1090
malt bread, 1 slice, 35g	19.9	+	0.8	94	399
naan, 1, 160g	80	3	20	538	2264
papadum, fried, 1, 13g	5.1	N	2.2	48	201
pitta, white, 1, 95g	55	2.1	1.1	252	1071
rye bread, 25g	11.4	1.1	0.4	55	233
soda bread, yeast-free, 1, 60g	35	1.2	1.5	178	750
toasted, regular, 1, 45g	19.5	1	0.5	93	390
tortillas made with wheat flour, 1, 30g	15	0.8	2	86	360
wheatgerm bread, 1 slice, 25g	10.9	0.8	0.8	57	244
white bread, average, 35g	17.3	0.5	0.7	82	357
white bread med. slice, large loaf, 36g	16.8	0.5	0.5	78	333
white bread roll, crusty, 1, 50g	28.8	0.8	1.1	140	596
white bread roll, soft, 1, 45g	23.2	0.7	1.9	121	512
white bread, fried in oil, 45g	21.8	0.7	14.3	226	946
white bread, with added fibre, 1 slice, 38g	17.4	1.1	0.5	81	342
wholemeal bread, average, 38g	15.8	2.2	0.9	82	347
wholemeal roll, 1 average, 48g	23.2	2.8	1.4	116	492
wholemeal, roll, 1 large, 105g	46	6	2.5	250	1050
stick, French (baguette), white, 1, 50g	22.5	0.7	1.5	128	540
stick, French (baguette), wholemeal, 1, 50g	21	+	1.5	119	500
toast, French, 2 slices	20	+	8.5	182	765
BROCCOLI					
raw, 100g	0	2.6	0	24	100
BRUSSELS SPROUTS					
raw, 100g	2	4.1	0	24	100

WHITE A good source of carbohydrate, fibre, vitamins and minerals. It contains less fibre than wholemeal varities, but is still low in fat and an important part of a healthy diet.

WHOLEMEAL AND MIXED GRAIN Both have more fibre and vitamins than white bread, with wholemeal having the most.

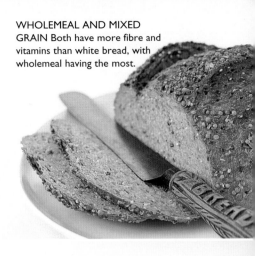

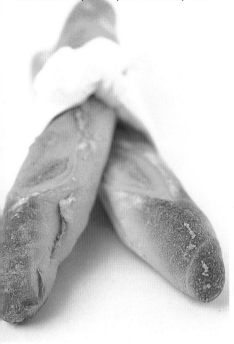

BREAD Let's dispel the myth once and for all that bread is fattening – it is the spreads that we cover it with that can be. Bread provides us with dietary fibre, energy and valuable vitamins and minerals, and even white bread is nutritious. One pitfall is that commercial bread can be high in sodium – check the label for details.

HI-FIBRE A flour with added fibre, which gives it the same amount of fibre as wholemeal. Perfect for school packed lunches.

RYE Light rye has a similar nutritional value to white bread, whereas dark or black rye is a better source of fibre, iron and magnesium.

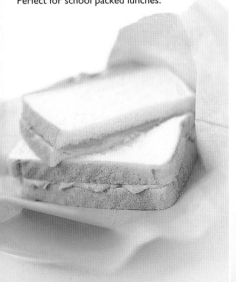

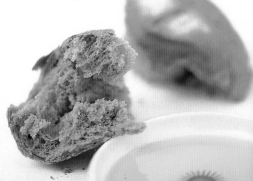

FOOD	CARB g	FIBRE g	FAT g	ENERGY kcal	ENERGY kJ
BUCKWHEAT KERNELS					
boiled, 100g	73	2.1	2.5	334	1400
BULGUR (Cracked Wheat)					
cooked, 100g	68.5	+	2.5	319	1340
BUN					
brioche, 1	N	N	16	278	1170
cinnamon, 1, 100g	45	1.5	15	263	1105
chelsea, 78g	43.8	1.3	10.8	285	1203
cream, 1 small, 60g	15.5	0.5	21.5	261	1082
finger, iced, 1, 65g	30	N	5	192	805
fruit, iced, 1, 90g	42	N	7	265	1115
hot cross, 1, 50g	29.3	1	3.5	155	657
BUTTER (see also FAT AND MARGARINE)					
clarified (ghee), 1tbsp	0	0	17	150	630
garlic, 1tbsp	0	0	16.5	145	610
regular, average, 1tbsp	0	0	16.5	145	610
reduced-fat average, 1tbsp	0	0	8	76	320
CABBAGE					
chinese, raw, 40g	0	0.6	0	3	14
chinese, flowering (pak choi), raw, 40g	0	1	0	5	20
mustard (dai gai choi), raw, 75g	0.5	2	0	11	45
red, raw, 40g	1	1.2	0	9.5	40
red, cooked, 60g	2	1	0	12	50
rolls, Lebanese, 3 small, 250g	40	+	10	290	1220
savoy, cooked, 60g	1	1.5	0	10	40
savoy, raw, 40g	1	1.5	0	7	30
CAKE					
angel, average slice	40.5	N	0.5	181	760
apricot crumble tea cake, 100g	44	+	15	324	1360
apple, average slice	40	+	10	252	1060
banana cake, 100g	68	+	16	428	1800
banana madeira, 100g	58	+	13.5	367	1540
banana tea loaf, 100g	57	+	12	351	1475
battenburg, 100g	50	N	17.5	370	1551
Bavarian chocolate, 100g	30	N	22.5	332	1395
black forest, 100g	40	N	17	331	1390
bran loaf, large slice, 100g	58.4	4.6	1.6	254	1081
cake mix, sponge, made up, 50g	27	N	8	280	1220
carrot cake, bought, 100g	44	+	23	402	1690
carrot cake, fingers, 100g	64	+	17	420	1770
cheesecake, 100g	30	0.4	20	320	1350
cherry cake, 100g	61.7	1.1	15.8	384	1657
chinese cakes, 100g	51.9	N	21.5	415	1740
chocolate, 100g	55	N	17	391	1645
christmas, 1 piece, 60g	33.5	+	6	193	810
coconut, 100g	51.2	2.5	23.8	434	1815
crispie cakes, 100g	73.1	0.3	18.6	464	1951
date loaf, 1 piece, 55g	27	+	4.5	158	665

BUTTER & MARGARINE

Which is healthier? In fact, they both have the same fat and calorie content, though margarines are usually lower in saturated fat than butter. Replacing butter, for example, with a polyunsaturated fat or monounsaturated spread may help reduce cholesterol levels in the blood. However, try to use all spreads sparingly.

DAIRY SPREADS Gaining in popularity, these spreads have some canola or olive oil added but they can still contain up to 42% saturated fat.

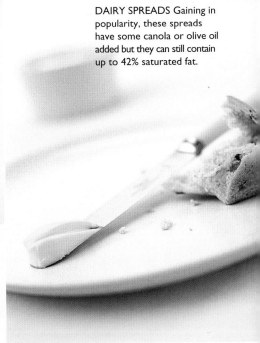

BUTTER By law, butter must contain over 80% fat. This fat is predominantly saturated and high in cholesterol.

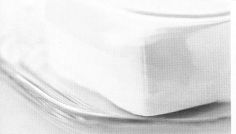

POLYUNSATURATED MARGARINES These are usually made with sunflower, safflower and soya bean oils. Replacing saturates in the diet with polyunsaturates may help lower blood cholesetrol levels. Some margarines that are high in polyunsaturates are now available in reduced-fat varieties.

REDUCED-FAT SPREADS A blend of milk fat or vegetable oil and water, with about 50% of the fat of butter or margarine.

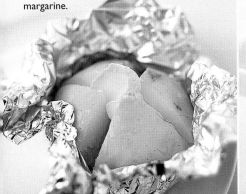

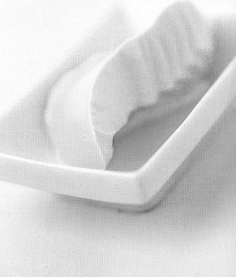

FOOD	CARB	FIBRE	FAT	ENERGY	
	g	g	g	kcal	kJ
CAKE CONT.					
date & walnut loaf, 1 piece, 60g	32	+	6	189	795
eclair, chocolate, bought, 70g	22.5	0.5	18	264	1110
flan, fruit, 100g	28.5	0.7	8	187	785
fruit, plain, 1 piece, 50g	271	+	6	165	695
fruit, retail, 1 piece, 70g	39	0.7	7	225	945
fruit cake, iced, 70g	43.9	1.2	8	249	1053
fruit cake, rich, 1 slice, 70g	41.7	1.2	7.7	239	1007
gateau, 1 slice, 85g	36.9	0.3	143	286	1201
gingerbread, 50g	32.4	0.6	6.3	190	800
hazelnut torte, average slice	N	+	30	402	1690
jam fairy, 100g	58.5	N	18	417	1750
jam sponge, 100g	67.5	1.8	2.5	312	1310
lamington, bought, 1, 75g	36	+	9	233	980
lamington, cream-filled, 1, 60g	30	+	7	187	785
lemon rolls, 100g	60.5	N	15	360	1510
madeira, 1 slice, 40g	23.4	0.4	6.8	157	661
madeira, iced, 100g	58	N	14	369	1550
marble, 100g	60	N	13.5	374	1570
mud, 100g	59	N	20	428	1800
rock, 1 medium, 60g	33	0.8	8	221	930
rum baba, average serving	47	N	10	326	1370
sponge cake, average slice, 60g	31.4	0.5	15.8	275	1152
sponge cake, fatless, 1 slice, 58g	30.7	0.5	3.5	171	722
sponge, fairy, 100g	60.5	N	8.5	344	1445
sponge, jam-filled, 1 slice, 60g	38.5	1.1	2.9	181	768
sponge with butter icing, slice, 60g	31.4	0.4	18.4	294	1228
swiss roll, 1 slice, 35g	22.5	0.5	2.5	114	480
swiss roll, chocolate, individual, 25g	14.5	N	2.8	84	355
CAPERS					
1 tbsp	1	+	0	7	30
CAPSICUM					
green, raw, 100g	2.5	1.6	0	15	65
red, raw, 100g	4	1.6	0	25	105
CAROB					
bar, 1, 45g	18	+	11.5	186	780
coated biscuit 1, 18g	9.5	N	5.5	89	375
powder, 2 tbsp, 40g	15	+	0	59	250
CARROT					
baby, raw, peeled, 50g	3	1.2	0	13	55
canned, 100g	4	1.9	0,	20	85
juice, 125ml	8	+	0	39	165
raw, peeled, boiled, 70g	4	2	0	19	80
CASSAVA peeled, boiled, 100g	30.5	1.6	0.5	131	550
CAULIFLOWER					
boiled, 100g	2	1.6	0	19	80
cheese, 200g	11	2	20	269	1130
raw, 50g	1	1	0	9	40

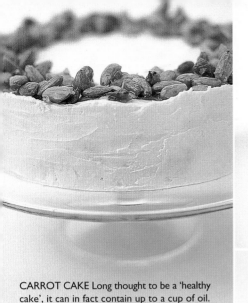

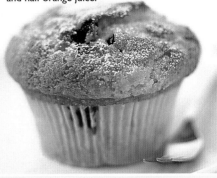

MUFFINS For healthy home-made muffins, use wholemeal self-raising flour to add fibre and replace the fat with half low-fat yoghurt and half orange juice.

CARROT CAKE Long thought to be a 'healthy cake', it can in fact contain up to a cup of oil. The cream cheese icing is high in fat and sugar.

RECIPE Fat-free sponge cake can be made by combining eggs, sugar, plain flour and baking powder. Add decoration and flavour with some high-fibre, sliced fruit.

CAKE As a general rule, the lighter and whiter the cake, the lower its fat content. Small amounts of any cake, as an occasional treat, can be eaten as part of a healthy diet. However, as a healthier option, go for fat-free sponge (see recipe) and fruit cakes (which contain more fibre) than creamy cakes with jam or butter icing. For increased fibre content, try making cakes with wholemeal flour.

SWISS ROLL A jam filling is less fattening than a cream one, though jam will increase the sugar content.

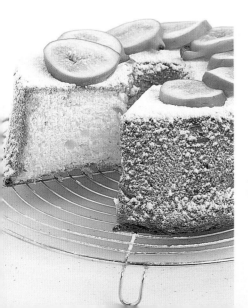

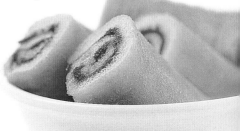

FOOD	CARB	FIBRE	FAT	ENERGY	
	g	g	g	kcal	kJ
CELERIAC					
fresh, Peeled, boiled, 100g	5.5	3.2	0	31	130
fresh, peeled, 120g	5	4.5	0	29	120
CELERY					
chopped, boiled, 63g	1.5	0.7	0	8	35
raw, 2 x 10cm sticks, 40g	1	0.5	0.5	5	20
CEREAL					
bran strands, 40g	18.6	9.8	1.4	104	444
bran with fruit and oats, 45g	34.5	9	1.5	138	580
bran, natural, 12g	7.5	4.5	0.5	33	140
bran, oat, unprocessed, 2 tbsp, 22g	11	3.5	1.5	53	225
bran, rice, 15g	7.5	4	3	70	295
bran, wheat, processed, 45g	31	14	2.5	161	675
bran, wheat, unprocessed, 2 tbsp, 10g	1	4	0.5	15	65
branflakes, 30g	20.8	3.9	0.6	95	406
chocolate flavoured rice pops, 30g	28.3	0.2	0.3	115	491
cornflakes, 30g	25.8	0.3	0.2	108	461
cornflakes, with nuts, 30g	26.6	0.2	1.2	119	507
crispies, rice based, 30g	27	0.2	0.3	111	472
crunchy oat bran flakes with fruit, 45g	31	N	2	160	675
crunchy oat bran flakes, 30g	22.2	3	1.2	107	456
fruit & fibre flakes, 30g	21.6	2.1	1.4	105	444
fruit & nut wheat flakes, 45g	31	3	1.5	157	660
grapenuts, 30g	25.5	+	1	113	475
high-energy multi flakes, 100g	81.7	2	1.7	355	1504
high-energy wheat flakes, 45g	35.5	2	1.5	170	715
high-protein rice flakes, 30g	24.5	0.6	0.3	113	481
honeynut cornflakes, 30g	26.6	0.2	1.2	119	507
honey wheat puffs, 30g	26.6	0.9	0.6	116	493
instant oats, 36g	24.7	2.6	2.8	134	569
muesli, swiss style, 50g	36.1	3.2	3	182	770
muesli with no added sugar, 50g	33.5	3.8	3.9	183	776
muesli, apricot & almond, 60g	35.5	+	4.5	210	880
muesli, apricot toasted, 30g	20	+	3	121	510
muesli, natural, 60g	39.5	2	2.5	208	875
muesli, oat & honey, 45g	31	+	7	188	790
muesli, traditional, 60g	37	2	4	221	930
muesli flakes, 45g	32	+	1	157	660
multigrain flakes, 30g	21.5	1	3	115	485
nut crunchie clusters, 45g	33.5	+	3.5	177	745
oat bran, crunchy, 45g	30	+	2.5	170	710
oat bran & fruit, 40g	30.5	+	3.5	168	705
oat flakes, 30g	23.5	+	1.5	115	485
porridge oats made with water, 200g	18	1.6	2.2	98	418
porridge, made with whole milk, 200g	27.4	1.6	10.2	232	976
puffed wheat, 20g	13.5	1.1	0.3	64	273
puffed wheat with honey, 30g	25.4	1	0.2	104	445
puffed wheat, sugar coated, 30g	25.4	1	0.2	104	445

CEREAL BRANS

Eating a healthy diet with plenty of fibre may help to prevent cancer of the bowel and constipation, and cereal brans (the husks of grain) are a concentrated source. However, uncooked bran contains phytates that hinder the absorption of minerals. The best way to boost your fibre intake is with wholegrain cereals and breads, legumes, fruit and vegetables.

HIGH-FIBRE BREAKFAST Packed with fibre, baked beans on a piece of wholemeal toast or muffin is a great start to the day.

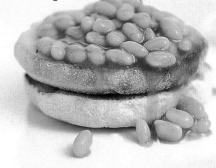
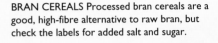

RECIPE Make a high-fibre smoothie by blending low-fat soya milk, yoghurt, a banana, honey and a tablespoon of oat bran.

BRAN CEREALS Processed bran cereals are a good, high-fibre alternative to raw bran, but check the labels for added salt and sugar.

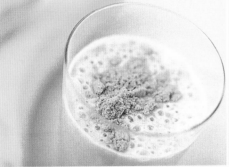
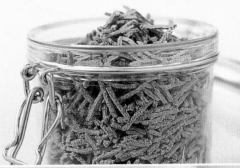

HOW MUCH? A tablespoon of bran provides a sixth of the recommended 30g of fibre a day. This is similar to the amount of fibre in a slice of wholemeal bread.

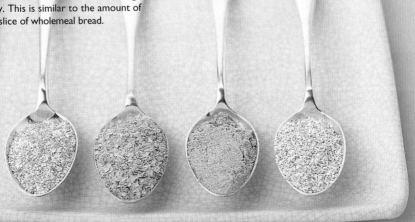

FOOD	CARB g	FIBRE g	FAT g	ENERGY kcal	ENERGY kJ

CEREAL CONT.

FOOD	CARB g	FIBRE g	FAT g	kcal	kJ
rice puffs, 30g	26.9	0.2	0.3	111	472
rice puffs, sugar coated, 30g	28.7	0.1	0.2	114	487
small whole wheat biscuits, 45g	33.3	4.3	0.7	149	635
small whole wheat biscuits with added fruit, 40g	30.2	3.2	0.8	135	573
sugar coated cornflakes, 30g	28.1	0.2	0.2	113	482
sultana bran flakes, 50g	34	5	0.8	150	645
wheat biscuits, 1, 20g	15	1.9	0.5	70	300
wheat flakes, 30g	24	2.6	0.8	108	459
wheat flakes and raisins, 40g	26	4	1.5	140	585
wheat rings, 100g	86.1	N	2.7	372	1581
wheat biscuits, 2, 40g	30	3.8	1	140	600
whole wheat biscuit, 1, 22g	15	2.2	0.7	72	304

CEREAL BAR (see also MUESLI BAR)

FOOD	CARB g	FIBRE g	FAT g	kcal	kJ
apricot fruity bar, 1 small	18	+	2.5	105	440
low sugar, 1 large	26	+	2.5	136	570
sports, 1	28.5	+	2.5	145	610

CHEESE

FOOD	CARB g	FIBRE g	FAT g	kcal	kJ
blue brie, 30g	0	0	13.5	126	530
blue castello, 30g	0	0	10	110	465
blue vein, 30g	0	0	9.5	110	465
bocconcini, 20g	0	0	7	76	320
brie, 30g	0	0	8.5	101	425
camembert, 30g	0	0	8	92	385
canola, mild, 30g	0	0	6.5	94	395
cheddar, 30g	0	0	10	122	505
cheddar, low-fat, 30g	0	0	7	99	410
cheddar, processed, 30g	0	0	8	99	415
cheddar, reduced-fat, 30g	0	0	7	98	410
cheddar slices, 20g	1	0	4.5	61	255
cheddar slices, reduced-fat, 20g	1	0	3	48	200
cheddar sticks, 20g	1	0	6	67	280
cheshire, 30g	0	0	10	114	480
cottage, 1tbsp	0	0	2	29	120
cottage, with cheese, 1tbsp	0.5	0	0.5	17	70
cottage, low-fat, 1tbsp	0.5	0	0.5	18	75
cottage with pineapple, low-fat, 1tbsp	3	0.5	0	27	115
creamed cottage, 1tbsp	0.5	0	1	24	100
creamed cottage, low-fat, 1tbsp	1	0	0.5	19	80
cream, 30g	1	0	10	101	425
cream, fruit, 30g	0	0	7.5	83	350
cream, light, 30g	1	0	5	48	200
cream, full fat, 30g	0.5	0	10	102	430
double Gloucester, 30g	0	0	10	120	505
edam, 30g	0	0	8	106	445
emmental, 30g	0	0	9	113	475
fetta, 30g	0	0	7	83	350
goat's, 30g	0.5	0	4.5	58	245

MUESLI This usually contains wheat and oat flakes with nuts and dried fruit. Choose varieties with no 'added' sugar. Muesli is high in fibre and a good source of many vitamins and minerals.

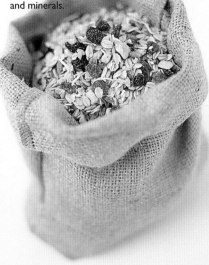

CEREAL Starchy foods such as breakfast cereals are an important part of a healthy diet. They provide carbohydrates, fibre and are often fortified with vitamins and minerals. However, it's best to avoid 'frosted' cereals or those containing 'added' sugar. Some cereals may also be high in fat and salt. Always check the label and try to choose wholegrain varieties.

SPORTS CEREALS Advertised as being the ideal way to begin your day, a lot of these are high in sugar, though relatively low in fat.

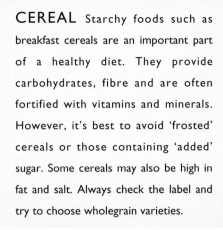

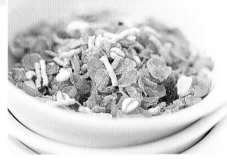

RECIPE If you love toasted muesli, try this low-fat version. Combine 2½ cups rolled oats, ½ cup oat bran and 175g mixed dried fruit and seeds. Drizzle with a very small amount of maple syrup and bake in a 180°C/350°F (Gas 4) oven for 20 minutes.

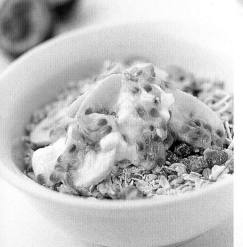

WHEAT BISCUITS These, together with other wholewheat cereals, are usually sugar free, low in fat and high in fibre. They make an excellent, filling start to the day.

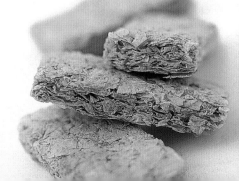

FOOD	CARB	FIBRE	FAT	ENERGY	
	g	g	g	kcal	kJ

CHEESE CONT.

gouda, 30g	0	0	9	113	475
halloumi, 30g	0	0	5	73	305
havarti, 30g	0	0	11	120	505
jarisberg, 30g	0	0	9	113	475
jarlsberg lite, 30g	0	0	5	82	346
lancashire, 30g	0	0	9.5	110	465
leicester, 30g	0	0	10	119	500
mozzarella, 30g	0	0	6.5	90	380
mozzarella, reduced-fat, 30g	0	0	5.5	86	360
parmesan, 30g	0	0	9.5	132	555
pizza, grated, 30g	0	0	6.5	93	390
processed, 30g	0	0	7	42	175
quark, 20g	0	0	2.5	26	110
quark, low-fat, 20g	0	0	0.5	15	65
reduced-fat, 20g	0	0	4.5	69	290
ricotta, 20g	0	0	2	30	125
ricotta, reduced-fat, 20g	0.5	0	1.5	25	105
ricotta, smooth, 20g	0	0	2	25	105
sheep's milk, fresh, 30g	0	0	6.5	90	380
soft, 30g	0	0	10	124	520
soya, 30g	0	0	8	93	390
stilton, 30g	0	0	9.5	111	465
swiss, 30g	0	0	9	114	480
wensleydale, 30g	0	0	9.5	112	470

CHERRIES

canned in syrup, drained, 100g	17	0.6	0	70	295
glace, 6, 30g	20	0.3	0	77	325
raw, weighed with stones, 100g	12	0.7	0.1	53	225

CHEWING GUM

sugarless, per piece, 10g	0	0	0	4	15
with sugar, per piece, 10g	3	0	0	9.5	40

CHICKEN

breast, no skin, grilled, 100g	0	0	5	157	660
breast, with skin, grilled, 100g	0	0	12.5	218	915
breast, quarter, no skin, barbecued, 100g	0	0	6	199	835
breast, quarter, with skin, rotisseried, 100g	N	0	12.5	214	900
breast, lean, 100g	0	0	1	40	170
chicken pastrami, 1 serving, 30g	N	N	1	40	170
crispy-skinned, 100g	0	0	3	64	270
drumstick, no skin, baked, 2	0	0	9	179	750
drumstick, with skin, baked, 2	0	0	14.5	229	960
drumstick crumbed, 145g	N	0	17	313	1315
fried chicken (see FAST FOOD)					
nuggets, 1, 20g	2.5	0	3.5	57	240

CHEESE Belonging in the milk and dairy food section of the food wheel (see page 14), cheese should be consumed in moderation. It is an excellent source of calcium – the mineral essential for healthy teeth and bones. Many cheeses are relatively high in fat, although reduced-fat varieties are becoming increasingly available.

COTTAGE CHEESE The winner in the low-fat competition. Buy the low-fat version and use as a spread, for dips or as a sandwich filling.

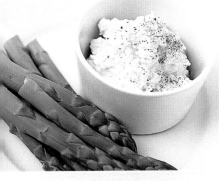

RICOTTA On average, this contains about 11% fat, compared to hard cheeses such as cheddar, which contain about 35% fat. However, although it is relatively low in fat, it is often used in popular Italian desserts, which aren't so healthy!

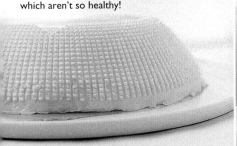

PARMESAN Hard cheeses can contain up to 35% fat, but with parmesan, the strong flavour means that, though high in fat, a little can go a long way. Grate with the fine side of the grater and you'll end up using less cheese.

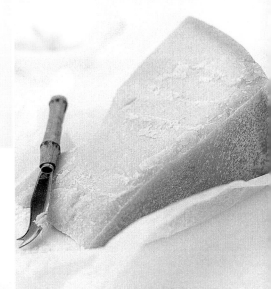

MOZZARELLA Pizza-lovers take note, this cheese is relatively high in fat (about 21%). If you're making pizza at home, replace half with low-fat mozzarella, so you get lots of taste, but less fat.

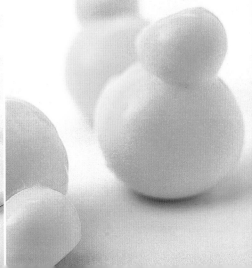

FOOD	CARB	FIBRE	FAT	ENERGY	
	g	g	g	kcal	kJ
CHICKEN CONT.					
roll, processed, 1 slice, 38g	4.5	N	9.5	158	665
sausage, cooked, skinless, 2	0	0	10	164	690
thigh, no skin, cooked, 2	0	0	6	126	530
thigh, with skin, cooked, 2	0	0	8	145	610
wing, with skin, cooked, 2	0	0	12	179	750
CHICKPEAS					
canned, drained, 186g	29.9	7.6	5.4	214	906
dried, boiled, 180g	32.8	7.7	3.8	218	922
CHICORY GREENS					
raw, 100g	2.8	1	0.6	11	45
CHILLI					
powder, 1 tsp, 5g	Tr	Tr	0	N	N
green, raw, each, 20g	1	N	0	4	15
red, raw, each, 20g	1	0.3	0	6	25
CHIVES					
fresh, 2 tbsp, 40g	Tr	0.8	0	1	5
CHOCOLATE					
after-dinner mint, 1, 6g	11	0	1.5	87	365
block, 100g	55.5	N	32.5	536	2250
coconut, bar, 1, 57g	33.2	+	14.9	270	1129
caramels, 1, 20g	12	0	5.5	99	415
cherry-flavoured centre,					
1, 55g	30.5	0	13.5	248	1040
cream, 100g	43	N	46.5	604	2535
cooking, dark, 100g	56	+	31	505	2120
cooking, milk, 100g	61.5	+	28.5	505	2120
coated wafer biscuits, 1, 45g	27	N	11.5	220	945
coated candies, 1 packet,					
55g	40	N	10.5	257	1080
coated peanuts, 1 packet,					
55g	34	+	13.5	273	1145
coated malt balls, 1 packet,					
45g	30	N	9.5	212	890
coated nougat and toffee bar,					
1, medium, 65g	43.2	+	12.3	285	1204
coated nougat bar, 1, 25g	13.5	N	9	137	575
coated whipped bar, 1, 26g	16.5	+	4.1	103	435
coated biscuit fruit and nut bar,					
1, 55g	27.5	+	16.5	280	1175
coated peanut bar, 1, 60g	36	+	13.5	283	1190
coated biscuit, 1, 55g	35	+	13.8	264	1128
choc bar, 1, 40g	23	+	11.5	204	855
full cream, milk, 1, 54g	32.1	+	16.4	286	1196
fruit & nut bar, 100g	54	+	34	540	2270
honeycomb bar, 80g	56	0	163	387	1625
in crisp sugar shells, 1 tube, 37g	27.3	+	6.5	169	711
soft centres, 100g	64.5	0	21.5	469	1970

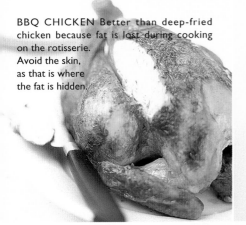

BBQ CHICKEN Better than deep-fried chicken because fat is lost during cooking on the rotisserie. Avoid the skin, as that is where the fat is hidden.

CHICKEN A good source of protein and B vitamins. If you are watching the amount of fat in your diet, avoid the skin of the chicken, which makes up about 50% of its fat content (remove it before cooking if possible). Without its skin, chicken is a low-fat source of protein, especially if you poach, steam or grill it.

RECIPE For a low-fat dinner, brush a skinless chicken breast or thigh fillet with a mixture of sweet chilli sauce, soy sauce and chopped fresh coriander. Barbecue or grill.

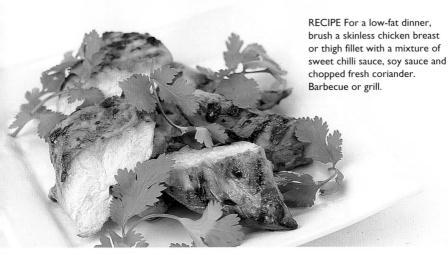

ROAST CHICKEN The juices that come out of a roasting chicken are high in saturated fat. Instead, place on a rack inside a pan and baste with a little oil.

BREASTS VS THIGHS Although chicken breast can be 2 or 3g lower in fat than the same amount of thigh meat, it tends to dry out if cooked for too long. Thighs are perfect for slower cooking in curries and casseroles.

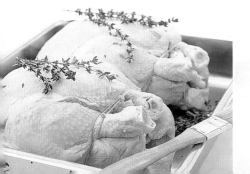

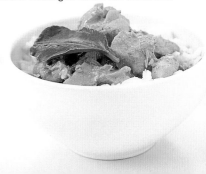

FOOD	CARB g	FIBRE g	FAT g	ENERGY kcal	kJ
CHOCOLATE CONT.					
triangular nougat bar, 1, 50g	28.5	N	15	264	1110
CHUTNEY					
fruit, homemade, 1tbsp	8.5	0.4	0	34	145
mango, 1tbsp	9	0.2	0	30	125
COCOA POWDER					
1tbsp	1.5	1.2	1	21	90
COCONUT					
cream, block,100g	7	+	68.8	669	2760
desiccated, dried, 25g	1.6	3.4	15.5	151	623
oil, 1tbsp	0	0	20	176	740
COFFEE					
for each teaspoon of sugar in coffee, add ...	5	0	0	19	80
cappuccino, whole milk, 1 cup, 200ml	N	0	5	89	375
cappuccino, skim milk, 1 cup, 200ml	N	0	0	50	210
decaffeinated, black,1 cup, 200ml	0	0	0	0	0
filtered, black, 1 cup, 200ml	Tr	0	0	7	30
ground, 1 cup + 25ml whole milk, 225ml	2.5	0	1	23	95
ground, 1 cup + 25ml skim milk, 225ml	2.5	0	0	18	75
iced, plain, 1 cup, 200ml	1.5	0	7	59	250
iced, with whole milk ice cream					
& cream, 325 ml	N	0	12	179	750
instant black, 1 cup, 200ml	0	0	0	2	8
instant, 1 cup + 25ml whole milk, 225ml	1.5	0	1	18	75
instant, 1 cup + 25ml skim milk, 225ml	1.5	0	0	13	55
Irish, 1 cup, 200ml	Tr	0	10	189	795
milk, 1tsp coffee + 1 cup whole milk, 200ml	12.5	0	10	173	725
mocha, 1 cup, 200ml	N	0	10	119	500
percolated, black, 1, cup, 200ml	Tr	0	0	0	0
whitener, 1tsp	2	0	1.5	21	90
CORDIAL (see also SOFT DRINKS)					
citrus, 25% juice, prepared, 1 glass, 250ml	17	0	0	65	275
citrus, 60% juice, prepared, 1 glass, 250ml	18	0	0	73	.305
citrus, reduced sugar					
lemon, prepared, 1 glass, 250ml	N	0	0	69	290
undiluted, 1tbsp	9	0	0	34	145
CORN					
baby, canned, 6, 100g	2	1.5	0.4	23	96
cob, 1, large, 100g	11.6	1.3	1.4	66	280
creamed, canned, 100g	20	+	1	81	340
kernels, canned, 30g	8	0.4	0.4	37	156
CORN CHIPS (see also SNACK FOOD)					
cheese, 40g	25.5	2	9.5	193	810
flavoured, 40g	20	2	12	198	830
toasted snacks, 40g	21.7	0.4	12.8	208	867
CORNMEAL dry, 40g	30	1	0.5	145	610
COUSCOUS cooked, 100g	23	+	0	112	470
CRABAPPLE raw, 60g	12	+	0	45	190

MILK CHOCOLATE This is usually made by adding milk solids to chocolate. It has the same sugar content as dark and white chocolate.

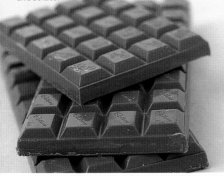

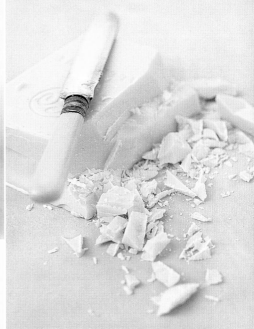

CHOCOLATE Good for an occasional energy boost, a chocolate bar is, however, high in fat and sugar and does contain caffeine. Chocolate is made up of about 30% fat, usually in the form of cocoa butter, and this is what gives chocolate its melt-in-the-mouth texture. Carob is also high in fat, although it is caffeine-free.

WHITE CHOCOLATE Not a true chocolate because it doesn't contain cocoa solids. It is, however, still made from cocoa butter, milk and sugar, and is high in fat.

DARK CHOCOLATE All chocolate is high in fat. However, high-quality chocolate has less sugar and, where this is the case, cocoa solids will come before sugar in the ingredients. Good-quality bitter chocolate has the least sugar.

COCOA The process of manufacturing cocoa powder removes much of the fat content (cocoa butter). Use in cooking to add chocolate flavour without too much fat.

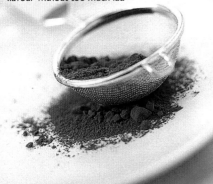

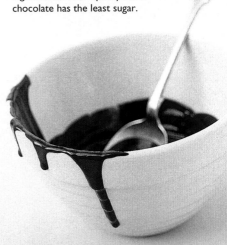

FOOD	CARB g	FIBRE g	FAT g	ENERGY kcal	kJ
CRACKERS (see also CRISPBREAD)					
cheese flavour, 2	4	+	1	24	100
cream, 2	4.5	0.4	2	40	170
rye, 2	5.5	1.6	1.5	38	160
rice snacks, cheese, 30g	22	+	2	117	490
rice snacks, sesame, 30g	22	+	2	117	490
sesame, 2	3	+	1	20	85
water crackers, 2	4.5	0.4	0.5	25	105
CRANBERRY JUICE 1 glass, 250ml	36.5	N	0	143	600
CREAM					
aerosol, whipped, 100ml	4	0	30.5	293	1230
clotted, 100ml	2	0	63	586	2413
crème fraîche, 100ml	2.5	0	48	440	1850
double thick, rich, 100ml	3	0	54.5	499	2095
light, 100ml	3.5	0	17.5	189	795
regular, 100ml	3	0	35.5	333	1400
thickened, 100ml	3.5	0	36.5	345	1450
thickened, light, 100ml	6	0	19	211	885
CREAM, SOUR					
extra light, 100ml	7	0	12.5	158	665
light, 100ml	5	0	18	193	810
regular, dairy 100ml	4	0	19	199	835
CREPE plain, 20g	7.5	0.5	2.5	65	275
CRISPBREAD					
high fibre, 1, 5g	4	1	0	17	70
bran & malt, 1	3.5	0.5	0	19	80
plain, 1	4.5	0.5	1	27	115
rye, 1, 10g	7.1	1.2	0.2	32	137
fat-free, 1	7	+	0	34	145
original, low fat, 1	5	+	1	32	135
puffed, 1	4	N	0	19	80
wholemeal, 1	5	+	1	29	120
swiss type, 1	16	1.2	0.5	79	330
— with sesame whole rye, 1	15	1.2	1	81	340
— multigrain, 1	9	1.2	1.5	60	250
— wholemeal, 1	9	1	1	58	245
wheatgerm type, original, 1	4	1	0.5	23	95
CROISSANT plain, 60g	23	1	12.2	216	903
CROUTONS 1 serving, 15g	11	1	1	61	255
CRUMPET					
regular, toasted, 40g	17.4	0.8	0.4	80	338
wholemeal, toasted, 45g	17	1.5	0.5	85	355
CUCUMBER					
lebanese, raw, unpeeled, 5 slices, 35g	1	0.5	0	4	15
raw, unpeeled, 5 slices, 45g	3	0.5	0	4	15
CUMQUAT (KUMQUAT)					
raw, peeled, 1, 20g	3	0.8	0	12	50
CURRANTS dried, 75g	50.9	1.4	0.3	200	854

RECIPE For a delicious low-fat alternative to cream, try combining low-fat ricotta with a little low-fat vanilla yoghurt.

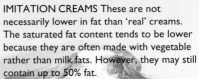
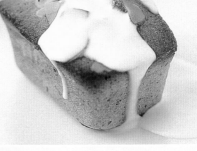

IMITATION CREAMS These are not necessarily lower in fat than 'real' creams. The saturated fat content tends to be lower because they are often made with vegetable rather than milk fats. However, they may still contain up to 50% fat.

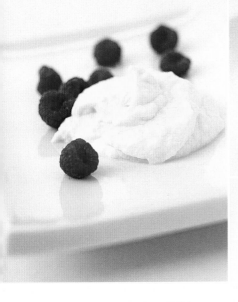

CREAM A concentrated source of saturated fat and calories. However, not all creams have the same fat content; a general rule is the thicker the cream, the higher the fat content. For example, single cream contains about 19% fat whereas clotted cream contains about 63% fat! Consider using low-fat yoghurt as a dessert alternative.

HALF-FAT CREAM This has about 13% fat – half that of full cream. However, if you use low-fat yoghurt as a substitute, you will reduce the fat level to just 1%.

EXTRA THICK CREAM Containing about 54% fat, this cream is a thick, rich and very indulgent treat

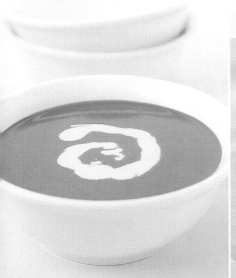

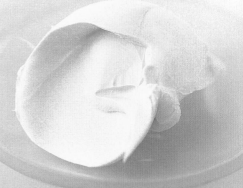

FOOD	CARB g	FIBRE g	FAT g	ENERGY kcal	kJ
CURRY PASTE					
curry paste, 1tbsp	1.5	N	2	24	100
curry powder 1tbsp	3	2.8	1.5	30	125
hot curry paste, 1tbsp	1.5	N	2	26	110
Indian, 1tbsp	5	0	9	98	410
tandoori, 1tbsp	2	0	0	49	205
CUSTARD					
baked, egg, 100ml	9	0	4.5	95	400
bread & butter custard, 100ml	15.5	0.5	5.5	132	555
custard & fruit, 100ml	16	+	1.5	86	360
powder, prepared with whole milk, 100ml	12.5	0	4	96	405
powder, prepared with reduced-fat milk 100ml	13.5	0	1.5	82	345
pouring, regular, 100ml	16	0	1.5	88	370
DANISH PASTRY					
almond, 100g	46	2	25	428	1800
apple, 100g	43.5	N	12	298	1250
apricot, 100g	38	N	12	270	1135
blueberry, 100g	40	N	12	286	1200
chocolate, 100g	24	N	19.5	280	1175
continental,100g	37.5	N	17	325	1365
custard, 100g	34.5	N	17	307	1290
pecan, 100g	52	N	20.5	417	1750
DATES					
dried, 6, 50g	28.5	2	0	113	485
fresh, seeded, chopped, 50g	14.5	0.9	0	54	228
DESSERT					
apple pie, bakery, 100g	28	+	8.5	198	830
apple pie, manufatured, 100g	38.5	1.7	12.5	279	1170
apple pie, reduced fat, 100g	32.5	+	7	199	835
apple & blackberry pie, 100g	42.5	+	17	336	1410
apple & rhubarb crumble, 120g	44	2	8	250	1050
apple strudel, 100g	41	+	11	273	1145
apricot pie, 100g	33	+	10	232	975
apricot pie, bought, 100g	38.5	+	14	293	1230
banana split with 3 scoops ice cream	55	1.1	10.5	325	1365
chocolate mocha, 100g	32.5	N	23.5	349	1465
bavarian, chocolate swirl, 100g	30.5	0	19.5	306	1285
blackberry & apple pie, 100g	35	+	10	232	975
chocolate mousse, 100g	28	0	13	232	975
chocolate mousse, dessert, 100g	23	0	9	201	845
chocolate mousse, light, 100g	19	0	4	136	570
Christmas pudding, 1 piece, 50g	29	1	6	167	700
custard tart 1, 135g	41	1.5	17.5	350	1470
junket (blancmange), 100g	48	0	3.5	114	480
lemon meringue pie, 1 piece, 75g	28.5	0.5	12.5	238	1000
pecan pie, 1 piece, 115g	64.5	+	21	450	1890
profiteroles, 1, 55g	N	+	9	130	545
pudding, blackberry sponge, 100g	59.9	+	5	299	1255

BACK-TO-BASICS Home-made rice custard or bread-and-butter pudding made with skimmed milk are great reduced-fat desserts.

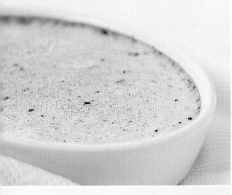

PIES AND TARTS The pastry in these tends to make them a high-fat option. Save them for occasional treats and choose fruit-based ones where possible.

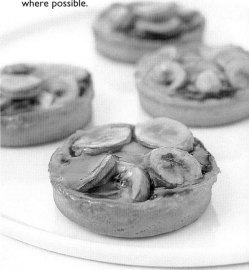

DESSERT

A sweet treat is a perfect way to end a meal, and it doesn't have to be high in fat. A fruit sorbet is a delicious dessert with no fat at all, while pancakes or puddings made with low-fat dairy products are full of energy-giving carbohydrates. Fruit, eaten on its own or with some low-fat yoghurt, is one of the tastiest and healthiest desserts of all.

RECIPE Bring 1 cup of low-calorie cordial, 4 cups of water and a cinnamon stick to the boil. Add a peeled pear and simmer for 10–15 minutes until tender. Serve with low-fat fromage frais.

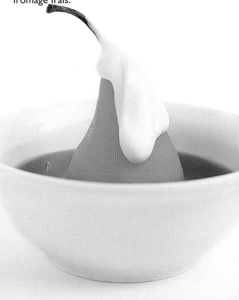

CANNED FRUITS Fruits cooked in their own juice rather than in a sugar syrup are lower in calories.

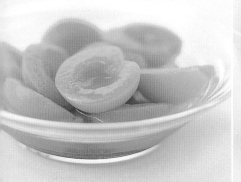

FOOD	CARB	FIBRE	FAT	ENERGY	
	g	g	g	kcal	kJ
DESSERTS CONT.					
pudding, bread & butter, 100g	N	0.3	10	299	1255
pudding, chocolate mousse, 100g	32	N	6	209	880
pudding, chocolate sponge, 100g	41.5	+	4	217	910
pudding, creme caramel, 100g	20	N	3	119	500
pudding, lemon sponge, 100g	41	+	3	204	855
pudding, plum, 60g	30	+	4.5	164	690
pudding, rice, banana, canned, 125g	N	+	13	244	1025
pudding, rice, canned, 150g	22.5	0.3	3.75	135	562
pudding, rice, chocolate, canned, 125g	N	+	6.5	209	880
souffle, 100g	10.5	N	14.5	200	840
tiramisu, 100g	N	N	20	328	1380
trifle, bought, 120g	33	0.5	7	209	880
DEVON split, 50g	3	+	9	117	490
DIPS					
barbecue, 1tbsp	2.5	0	4.5	51	215
chicken & asparagus, 1tbsp	2	0	3	40	170
chilli, chip & dip type, 1tbsp	1.5	N	0	8	35
chive & onion, 1tbsp	1	0	6.5	65	275
chunky bean, 1tbsp	2.5	+	0	11	45
corn & bacon, 1tbsp	2	+	1	20	85
corn relish, 1tbsp	2	0	3	37	155
cucumber & yoghurt, 1tbsp	0	+	2	26	110
French onion, reduced fat, 1tbsp	1	0	3.5	43	180
French onion, average, 1tbsp	0	0	5	61	255
French onion, low-fat, 1tbsp	3	0	2.5	42	175
gherkin dip, 1tbsp	3	+	4	49	205
herb & garlic, 1tbsp	2	+	4	45	190
hot & spicy, 1tbsp	2	0	3.5	44	185
hummus, 1tbsp	2	0.6	3.5	45	190
taramasalata, 1tbsp	2	+	4	46	195
DOLMADES 60g	14.5	+	4	101	425
DOUGHNUT					
cinnamon sugar, 1 large, 75g	36.6	+	10.9	252	1061
cream-filled, 1, 70g	21	+	17	251	1055
iced, 1, 80g	38.5	+	19.5	339	1425
DRESSINGS (see also MAYONNAISE)					
caesar, 1tbsp	3	0	7	76	320
caesar, creamy, 1tbsp	2	0	7	70	295
coleslaw, average, 1tbsp	7	0	7	88	370
coleslaw, reduced fat, 1tbsp	5	0	7	82	345
coleslaw, light, 1tbsp	5.5	0	3.5	57	240
French, 1tbsp	2.5	0	4.5	49	205
French, olive oil, 1tbsp	3	0	3.5	43	180
French, low-fat, 1tbsp	3.5	0	0	14	60
Italian, 1tbsp	1.5	0	6	59	250
Italian, light, 1tbsp	2	0	3.5	40	170
Italian, low fat, 1tbsp	3.1	0	0	12	50

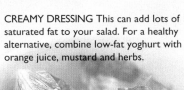

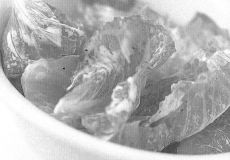

CREAMY DRESSING This can add lots of saturated fat to your salad. For a healthy alternative, combine low-fat yoghurt with orange juice, mustard and herbs.

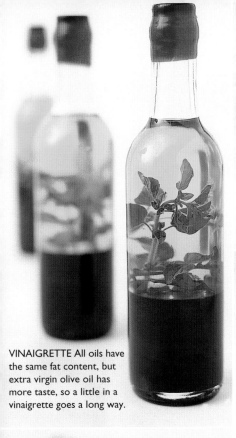

VINAIGRETTE All oils have the same fat content, but extra virgin olive oil has more taste, so a little in a vinaigrette goes a long way.

DRESSINGS

A green salad is packed with fibre, vitamins and minerals, but a heavy hand with the dressing can add lots of unwanted calories. However, the vegetable oils in most dressings contain the more healthy monounsaturated or polyunsaturated fats, as well as vitamin E. Use more juice or vinegar to oil for a zesty dressing with less fat.

RECIPE Make a low-fat juice dressing by combining orange juice, mustard, honey and a very small amount of olive oil.

SIMPLE DRESSING Avocados contain quite a lot of fat. Instead of an oily dressing, try just a squeeze of lemon juice and some black pepper.

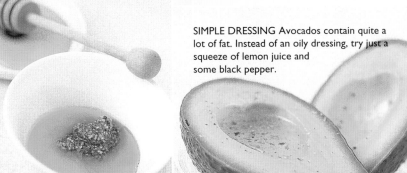

FOOD	CARB g	FIBRE g	FAT g	ENERGY kcal	kJ
DRESSINGS CONT.					
lemon pepper, reduced fat, 1tbsp	5	0	2	37	155
potato salad, 1tbsp	2.5	0	7	76	320
thousand island, 1tbsp	3.5	0	7	76	320
thousand island, light, 1tbsp	3.5	0	4	51	215
DRINKING POWDER					
barley type milk drink, 1tbsp	6	N	0	31	130
bournvita, 1tbsp	1.5	N	0	24	100
cocoa, 1tbsp	1.5	1.2	1	21	90
diet hot chocolate mix, 1 sachet	7	N	1	44	185
malted milk drink, 1tbsp	8	Tr	0	38	160
milk, 1tbsp	5.5	0	0.5	32	135
milkshake, strawberry, 1tbsp	12	0	0	50	210
Swiss style diet hot chocolate mix, 1 sachet	4	N	0	20	85
DUCK					
roast, no skin, 100g	0	0	9.5	182	765
roast, skin, 100g	0	0	26	307	1290
EGG					
1 small, 45g	0	0	4.5	64	270
1 medium, 55g	0	0	5.5	77	325
1 large, 60g	0	0	6	84	355
boiled 1, 53g	0	0	5.5	80	335
duck, boiled, 1, 65g	Tr	0	9	114	480
eggs benedict, 2 eggs	0	N	52	690	2900
fried, 1, 60g	0	0	8	98	410
fried, 2 × 60g, with 1 lean grilled bacon rasher	Tr	0	19	251	1055
omelette, plain or herb, 2 × 60g eggs	0	0	17	214	900
poached, 1, 60g	0	0	6	76	320
poached, 2 × 60g, with lean grilled bacon rasher	Tr	0	16	236	990
quail, raw, 1, 10g	0	0	1	15	65
replacer, 1tsp	1.5	0	1	31	130
scrambled, 2 × 60g	Tr	0	16	195	820
turkey, raw, 1, 80g	Tr	0	9.5	134	565
white only, 1, 31g	0	0	0	14	60
yolk only, 1	0	0	5	54	225
EGGPLANT (see also AUBERGINE)					
baby, 4, 65g	1.5	1.5	0	11	45
fried in oil, 100g	2.8	2.3	32	302	1262
grilled, 3 slices, 90g	2.5	2	0	18	75
raw, 100g	2.2	2	0.4	15	64
ELDERBERRIES raw, 145g	10.5	++	0.5	51	215
ENDIVE					
Belgian, raw, 60g	0	1.2	0	6	25
curly, 80g	0	1.6	0	6	25
FALAFEL commercial, 2, 60g	10	+	9	140	590
FAST FOOD (SHOP BOUGHT)					
apple pie, 1, 80g	30.5	1.3	13	239	1005
bacon & cheese chicken fillet burger, 190g	34.5	+	22.2	460	1930

EGG A good source of protein, vitamins and minerals, eggs have had a hard time because of fears about their high cholesterol level. In fact, to keep your blood cholesterol low, it is more important to avoid saturated fat in your diet. So providing they are eaten in moderation, eggs can form part of a nutritious diet.

SATURATED FAT Eggs contains about 10% fat, of which under half is saturated. The healthiest way to cook an egg is by boiling or poaching it.

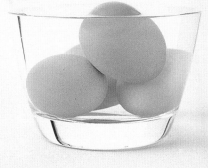

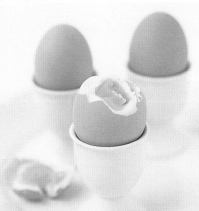

EGG YOLK Very nutritious, but also the source of cholesterol and fat in an egg.

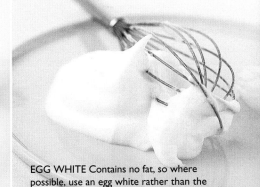

EGG WHITE Contains no fat, so where possible, use an egg white rather than the whole egg.

RECIPE Make a reduced fat omelette by using one whole egg, 2 egg whites and some skimmed milk. Mix in fresh herbs and cook without fat in a non-stick pan.

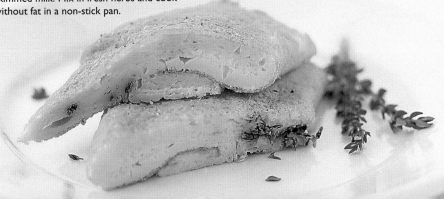

FOOD	CARB	FIBRE	FAT	ENERGY	
	g	g	g	kcal	kJ

FAST FOOD (SHOP BOUGHT) CONT.

FOOD	CARB	FIBRE	FAT	kcal	kJ
bacon & cheese burger, 1, 213g	52	+	18.3	487	2045
big burger, 1, 345g	55	+	32	646	2715
chips, regular, 117g	33	2.2	20	327	1375
chips, thick cut, 95g	25	2	13	233	980
chips, thin, 110g	37.4	2.3	17	308	1291
chicken nuggets, 7, 133g	17.5	+	29.5	411	1725
chicken nuggets, 4, 76g	10	+	17	236	990
chicken fillet burger, 1, 160g	28	+	16.5	282	1185
coleslaw, small tub, 116g	16	+	7	129	540
corn, 1 cobette, 78g	17	1.1	1	89	375
cornish pastie, 1, 155g	48	1.4	31.6	515	2151
fish, battered & deep-fried, 1 fillet, 145g	20	0.6	23	365	1535
fish stick, crab-flavoured, fried, 1, 27g	3.5	0	1.5	38	160
frankfurters, boiled, 2, 100g	3.5	+	20	247	1040
french fries, small, 76g	28.5	1.5	12	226	950
french fries, regular, 114g	42.5	2.3	18	337	1415
french fries, large, 159g	59	3	25	470	1975
fried chicken, coated, 2 pieces, 154g	8.5	+	29	413	1735
grilled chicken burger, 1, 180g	43.5	+	20	484	2035
hamburger, plain, 1, 170g	38	+	17.5	379	1590
hamburger, with bacon, 1, 185g	40.5	+	24	467	1960
hamburger, with cheese, 1, 195g	41.5	+	26	501	2105
hamburger, with egg, 1, 220g	44	+	26	517	2170
hot dog, 1, 100g	18.5	+	15	246	1035
individual cheesecake, 75g	25	0.3	7	175	735
individual chocolate mousse, 75g	17	N	5.5	132	555
mashed potato & gravy, small tub, 120g	12.5	+	2	80	335
nuggets, 6 pieces, 106g	18.5	+	16.5	276	1160
sundae, caramel/chocolate, 1, 141g	36	0	9	240	1010
sundae, strawberry, 1, 141g	36	0	6.5	218	915
thickshake, average, all flavours, 1, 240g	48.5	0	8	299	1255

FAST FOOD (TAKE-AWAY)

FOOD	CARB	FIBRE	FAT	kcal	kJ
apple pie, 1, individual, 100g	56.7	1.7	15.5	369	1554
bacon and egg muffin, 1, 145g	32.5	+	19.5	377	1585
big breakfast, 1, 250g	475	+	31	568	2385
big burger in bun, 1, 205g	40	+	30	562	2360
cheeseburger, 1, 122g	33	+	12.5	300	1260
chicken nuggets, 9 pieces, 171g	26	+	26.5	212	890
cookies, 1 box	47	+	8.5	274	1150
fillet-of-fish, 1, 146g	40	N	16	351	1475
french fries, small	37.4	2.3	17	308	1291
french fries, medium	52	3.2	22.5	414	1740
french fries, large	65	4	30	527	2215
fried chicken, 1, 184g	46	0	20.5	424	1780
hash browns, 1, 54g	15	1.5	7	124	520
hot cakes, with butter & syrup, 1 serving	85	N	15	479	2010
junior burger, 1, 100g	30	N	10	267	1120

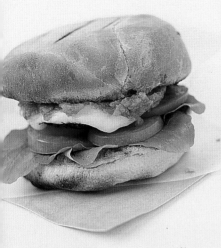

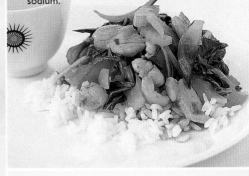

CHINESE Not too bad if you like stir-fries, but deep-fried or battered dishes are fattening. Accompany your meal with steamed rice, not fried, and note that soy sauce is high in sodium.

HAMBURGER This can be nutritious if home-made with lean mince, lettuce and tomato. If you're getting a take-away, skipping the cheese can cut the fat intake by about a third.

FAST FOOD

Today, more and more people are taking advantage of take-away food. It can be high in fat but, if you look carefully, you'll find there are healthy options. A side dish of vegetables or a salad will fill you up and should be low in fat, providing it doesn't come with lashings of dressing. Choose chunky bread for sandwiches with low-fat fillings.

PIES These are generally very high in fat, especially saturated fat – even if the filling isn't meat. Try to keep your consumption of pies and pastries to a minimum.

THAI Noodle and some stir-fried dishes are a healthy choice. Avoid curries made with coconut milk as it is high in saturated fat.

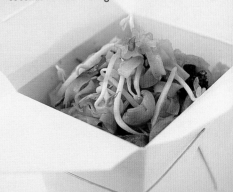

FOOD	CARB	FIBRE	FAT	ENERGY	
	g	g	g	kcal	kJ

FAST FOOD CONT.

FOOD	CARB	FIBRE	FAT	ENERGY	
pan pizza, cheese, 1 slice, 105g	24.8	1.5	11.8	235	984
pan pizza, hawaiian, 1 slice, 125g	35	2	11	292	1225
pan pizza, premium range, 1 slice, 143g	35.5	2.5	15	339	1425
pan pizza, extra topping, 1 slice, 136g	32	2	16	342	1435
pizza thin crispy base, cheese, 1 slice, 79g	21.5	1.5	9	217	910
pizza thin crispy base, hawaiian, 1 slice, 99g	26	2	9.5	242	1015
pizza thin crispy base, premium type, 1 slice, 114g	25.5	2	14	289	1215
pizza thin, crispy base, extra topping, 1 slice, 114g	27	2.5	12.5	286	1200
quarter pounder burger, no cheese, 1, 176g	36	+	19.5	417	1750
sausage & egg muffin, 1, 162g	32	+	22	412	1730
sundae, hot caramel, 1, 175g	56.5	0	8	311	1305
sundae, hot fudge, 1, 175g	50	0	11	319	1340
sundae, strawberry, 1, 171g	47	Tr	6	255	1070
sundae, without topping, 1, 134g	29	0	6	183	770
samosa, meat, commercial, heated, 3, 45g	14	1	9	145	610
sausage roll, 1, 130g	31.5	1.5	23	371	1560
spring roll, deep-fried, 1 large, 175g	48	2	17	398	1670
thickshake, chocolate, regular, 1, 305g	60	+	9.5	360	1510
thickshake, strawberry, large, 1 , 419g	81	0	12.5	480	2015

FAT (see also BUTTER AND FAT)

FOOD	CARB	FIBRE	FAT	ENERGY	
cocoa butter, 1tbsp	0	0	20	176	740
dripping, 1tbsp	0	0	20	176	740
lard, 1tbsp	0	0	20	176	740
replacer, 1tbsp	0	0	0	75	315
shortening, 1tbsp	0	0	16	143	600
suet, 1tbsp	Tr	0	17.5	162	680

FENNEL

FOOD	CARB	FIBRE	FAT	ENERGY	
raw, 1 bulb, 150g	5	3.6	0	18	75
steamed, 1 bulb, 150g	5.5	3.4	0	16	70

FIGS

FOOD	CARB	FIBRE	FAT	ENERGY	
dried, 5, 75g	40	5.6	1.2	40	168
ready to eat, 30g	14	2	0.5	63	267
raw, 1, 40g	4	0.6	0	17	74
stewed, sweetened, 100g	34	3.9	0.8	143	612

FISH (see SEAFOOD)

FLOUR

FOOD	CARB	FIBRE	FAT	ENERGY	
arrowroot, 100g	94	0.1	0.1	355	1515
barley, 100g	74.5	+	1.5	344	1445
besan, chickpea, 100g	49.6	10.7	5.4	313	1328
buckwheat, 100g	76.3	2.1	1.5	364	1522
corn, 100g	92	0.1	0.7	354	1508
maize, 100g	76	+	4	363	1525
millet, 100g	75.4	N	1.7	354	1481
potato, 100g	80	5.7	0.5	329	1380
rice, 100g	80.1	2	0.8	366	1531

FISH AND CHIPS Remember that the thinner the chips, the larger the surface area, and so more fat is absorbed during frying. Try grilled fish instead of battered. Bear in mind that spring rolls, battered savs and dim sims are all high in saturated fat.

PIZZA Salami, ham and cheese are all high-fat toppings, but any pizza without cheese or meat should be a good choice. If your pizza has a filled base, that'll add calories.

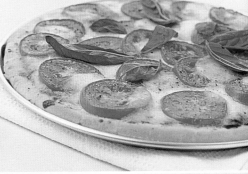

FAST FOOD The occasional take-away meal or snack is fine if you usually eat a balanced diet. Fast food tends to be short on fresh fruit and vegetables, so a vegetarian pizza or stir-fry would be a good choice, or make up for it later in the day with a low-fat, high-fibre meal that includes an extra portion of vegetables or fruit.

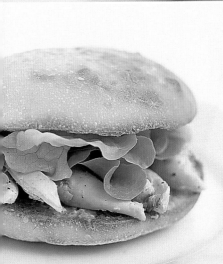

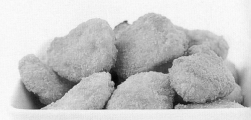

SKIN-FREE CHICKEN A lot of the fat in chicken is in the skin, so skin-free chicken is a good choice for a low-fat sandwich or burger.

CHICKEN NUGGETS For a low-fat version of these tasty snacks, cut chicken fillets into bite-size pieces, toss in egg white, then coat with cornflake crumbs. Bake in a 200°C (400°F/Gas 6) oven for 10–12 minutes.

FOOD	CARB g	FIBRE g	FAT g	ENERGY kcal	kJ
FLOUR CONT.					
rye, wholemeal, 100g	75.9	11.7	2	335	1428
semolina, raw, 100g	77.5	1.2	1.8	350	1489
soya, full-fat, 100g	23.5	11.2	23.5	447	1871
soya, low-fat 100g	28.2	13.5	7.2	352	1488
wheat, white, plain, 100g	77.7	3.1	1.3	341	1450
wheat, white, self-raising, 100g	75.6	3.1	1.2	330	1407
wheat, wholemeal, plain, 100g	63.9	9	2.2	310	1318
FRANKFURTER					
canned, drained, cooked, 175g	1.5	N	13	155	650
cocktail, canned. cooked, 1, 30g	0.5	0	5	62	260
cocktail, fresh, cooked, 1, 30g	1	N	6	74	310
fresh, cooked, 1, 75g	2.5	N	15	186	780
FRITTATA					
courgette & spinach, 1 slice, 250g	2	+	38.5	434	1825
Spanish (potato), 1 slice, 250g	13.5	+	27.5	369	1550
FROGS LEGS 2 fried	0	0	10	178	750
FROMAGE FRAIS					
apricot, honey & vanilla, 130g	20	0	0.5	118	495
orange tangerine, 130g	20	0	0.5	120	505
peach & mango, 130g	14.5	0	5	113	475
strawberry, 130g	15	0	5	115	485
strawberry, light, 130g	18	0	0.5	111	465
vanilla, 130g	15	0	5	115	485
vanilla, light 130g	29	0	6	230	965
petit pot, 60g	10	0	5	87	365
FROZEN DINNERS					
beef goulash, 400g	57	N	10	409	1720
beef hot-pot, 400g	39	N	11	356	1495
beef, healthy eating type, 310g	37	+	8	277	1165
bubble & squeak, 1 serving	8.5	0	2	51	215
chicken carbonara, low fat, 400g	76	N	11.5	424	1780
chicken chasseur, healthy eating type, 310g	34	+	3.5	251	1055
chicken tikka, healthy eating type, 400g	56	N	11	390	1640
curried prawns, 350g	53	N	4.6	299	1255
fettucine carbonara, 375g	49	N	30.8	552	2320
fettucine mediterranean, healthy eating type, 400g	58	N	11	395	1660
fillet of lamb, healthy eating type, 310g	9	+	8	236	990
fish fingers, grilled, 375g	15	0.5	7.5	155	650
French style chicken, low fat variety, 400g	72	N	11.5	486	2040
fried rice, 350g	20	N	7.5	390	1640
Indian style chicken, low fat, 400g	64	N	11	448	1880
roast pork, healthy eating type, 320g	34	N	5.5	277	1165
lamb, low fat, 400g	64	N	10	419	1760
shepherd's pie, 170g	13.5	1.5	8	177	745
Thai style chicken curry, low fat, 400g	64	N	12	438	1840
veal cordon bleu, healthy eating type, 320g	47	N	29	515	2165

WHITE FLOUR For those who really don't like wholemeal flour, white flour can still be nutritious and is a good protein source.

RICE FLOUR This is a good alternative to wheat flour for anyone with a gluten-intolerance. Maize cornflour, soya and potato flour are also gluten-free.

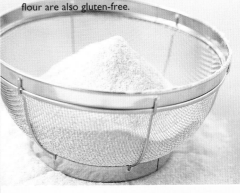

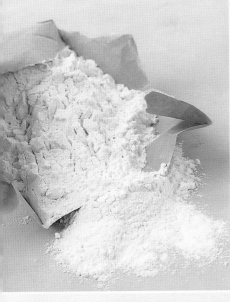

FLOUR Made into breads, cakes, biscuits and pasta, flour is a good source of carbohydrate. Wholemeal flour is made from the whole grain, while white flour is made after the husk of the grain has been removed and, though still nutritious, does have less fibre, vitamins and minerals. Self-raising flour has more sodium than plain flour.

WHOLEMEAL Full of fibre, vitamins and minerals, wholemeal flour can be used wherever you'd use white flour in cakes, breads, biscuits and pasta-making (you may need to add a little extra water).

SOYA A strong, gluten-free flour that is a richer source of protein than most flours. It can be combined with other flours to make batters and breads.

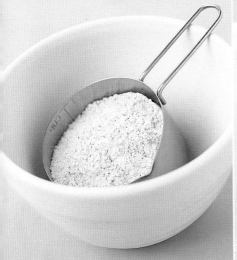

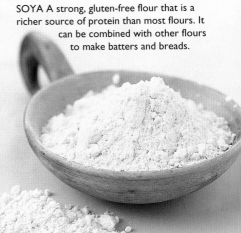

FOOD	CARB g	FIBRE g	FAT g	ENERGY kcal	kJ
FRUIT (see INDIVIDUAL FRUITS)					
FRUIT BAR					
fruit fingers, apricot/strawberry/					
tropical, 1, 22g	15	1	0.5	74	310
fruit fingers, raspberry, 1 bar, 15.6g	13	+	0.5	58	245
fruit roll, 1 bar, 37.5g	23	+	2	162	680
FRUIT, DRIED (see INDIVIDUAL FRUITS)					
FRUIT SALAD (see also INDIVIDUAL FRUITS)					
canned in pear juice, drained,					
1 bowl, 220g	20.5	3.5	0	92	385
canned in syrup, drained, 1 bowl, 220g	25.5	2.5	0	106	445
fresh, 1 bowl, 140g	19.3	2.1	0.1	77	332
GARLIC					
fresh, 2 peeled cloves, 6g	0.5	+	0	6	25
powder, 1tbsp	7.5	0	0	13	55
puree, 1tbsp, 15g	2.5	N	5	57	236
GELATINE 1tbsp	0	0	0	42	175
GHERKINS drained, 36g	9	0.4	0	38	160
GINGER					
beer, dry, 1 cup, 250ml	22	0	0	82	345
gingerbread biscuit, large, figure type, 70g	34.5	1	11.5	249	1045
ground, 1tbsp	4	+	0.5	19	80
raw, peeled, grated, 1tbsp	0.5	N	0	4	15
GNOCCHI					
potato/pumpkin, average serving, 150g	13	N	12	213	895
GOLDEN SYRUP 1tbsp	21.5	0	0	83	350
GOOSE lean, roast, 100g	0	0	23	315	1325
GOOSEBERRIES					
canned, in syrup, 100g	18.5	1.7	0.2	73	310
raw, 100g	3	2.4	0	19	81
GOURD					
bottle, raw, peeled, 75g	0.6	1.9	0	8	35
ridge, raw, peeled, 75g	N	1.5	0	13	55
wax, raw, peeled, 75g	1	1	0	4	15
GRAPEFRUIT					
canned in juice, 125g	19	0.5	0	78	330
juice, sweetened, 1 glass, 200ml	19	0	0	87	365
juice, unsweetened, 1 glass, 200ml	16	0	0	71	300
raw, peeled, 1/2 whole, 110g	5	1	0	27	115
GRAPES					
black, 100g	15	0.7	0	63	265
black, muscatel, 100g	19	0.7	0	78	330
green, 100g	12.5	0.7	0	56	235
green, sultana, 100g	15	0.7	0	61	255
juice, sweetened, 1 glass, 200ml	N	0	1	84	355
juice, unsweetened, 1 glass, 200ml	N	0	1	84	355
GRAVY POWDER dry, 1tbsp	8	0	0.5	39	165
prepared, 225g	3	0	0	14	60

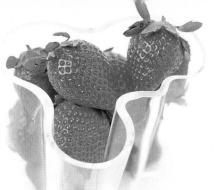

BERRIES A rich source of Vitamin C, all berries contain anitoxidants and they are also low in calories.

FRUIT Packed with vitamins and fibre, fruit is also low in fat and calories. According to healthy guidelines, we should all aim to eat at least five portions of fruit and vegetables every day. Choose from a variety of fresh, dried, canned (in natural juice rather than syrup) and frozen. Fruits are also rich in antioxidants (see Food Terms).

APPLE A good source of Vitamin C and fibre, apples make a cheap, convenient, healthy snack for between meals.

PAWPAW/PAPAYA Half a medium pawpaw contains lots of beta carotene (an antioxidant) and twice the daily requirement of Vitamin C.

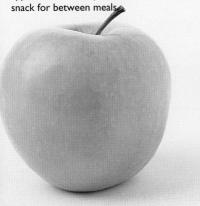

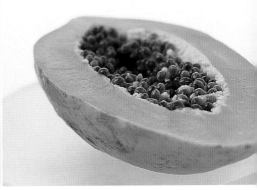

DRIED FRUITS A rich source of dietary fibre, potassium and some iron, dried fruits don't contain much vitamin C. They can also be high in 'natural' fruit sugar—fructose, which causes tooth decay in the same way as sugar.

RECIPE Place some dried fruit in a pan, cover with apple or orange juice and bring to the boil. Stand for 15 minutes until the fruit is plump, then serve warm with low-fat yoghurt.

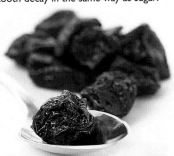

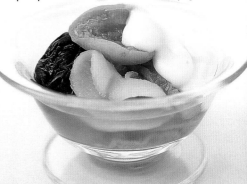

FOOD	CARB	FIBRE	FAT	ENERGY	
	g	g	g	kcal	kJ
GUAVA					
canned in juice, 100g	15.7	3	0	60	258
raw, 1 medium, 100g	5	3.7	0.5	26	112
HAGGIS boiled, 100g	19.2	N	21.7	310	1292
HALVA 30g	14.5	+	5	102	430
HAM					
& chicken luncheon meat, 2 slices, 23g	1	N	4	53	225
leg, canned, 2 slices, 35g	0	0	1.5	39	165
leg, fresh, lean, 2 slices, 46g	0	0	1.5	50	210
leg, fresh, untrimmed, 2. slices, 50g	0	0	4	70	295
light, 90% fat-free, 2 slices, 50g	0	0	2.5	36	150
shoulder, 2 slices, 50g	0	0	3	55	230
shoulder, canned, 2 slices, 35g	0	0	2	42	175
steak, grilled, 1, 115g	0	0	9	186	780
HAMBURGER (see FAST FOOD)					
HERBS					
average all varieties, dried, 1tbsp	Tr	N	0	19	80
average all varieties, fresh, chopped, 1tbsp	Tr	N	0	17	70
HONEY 1tbsp	22	0	0	84	355
HONEYCOMB 1 piece, 30g	22.2	0	1.5	86	360
HORSERADISH					
cream, 1tbsp	2.5	0.2	2	32	135
fresh, 5g	0.5	0.3	0.5	8	35
HUMMUS average serving, 100g	11.6	2.4	12.6	187	781
ICE CREAM BLOCK					
chocolate, 1, 158ml	36.5	0	0	150	630
neopolitan, 100ml	20	0	0	88	370
fruit-flavoured, 100ml	12.5	0	1	67	280
ICE CREAM					
caramel, 1	18	0	6	133	560
chocolate bar type, 1	21	0	19	260	1090
chocolate, 100ml	23	0	11.5	208	875
cone, large, vanilla,. 1, 70g	24	0	12.5	220	925
cone, chocolate, 1, 70g	23	0	13.5	226	950
cone, single, plain wafer type, 1, 15g	4	0	0	19	80
cone, sugar, 1, 10g	8.5	0	0.5	40	170
cone, waffle, 1, 18g	3.5	0	0	15	65
cone with 1 small scoop ice cream	8.5	0	3	64	270
cone with 1 small scoop reduced-fat ice cream	8.5	0	1.5	54	225
fruits of the forest, 1, 86ml	20	0	6	142	595
lemon, 86ml	18.5	0	6	137	575
mango, 100ml	21	0	8	168	705
raspberry, 1, 90ml	17.5	0	3.5	107	450
soft-serve, 1, 100ml	21.5	0	4.5	137	575
stick, chocolate flavoured, 1, 90ml	19	0	3.5	126	530
stick, vanilla, chocolate coated, 1, 93ml	20.5	0	17.5	248	1040
stick, Belgian chocolate coated ice cream 1, 120ml	43	0	27	432	1815
tub, fruit cream, 100ml	10	+	5	94	395

HERBS Adding herbs to your food is a healthy way to enhance the flavour of dishes without loading on the fat and salt. Many people also claim that herbs have medicinal properties and many of today's medical drugs do indeed come from plants. If you are interested in herbal medicine, try some herbal teas, which are now widely available.

BASIL Delicious with tomato dishes and the essential ingredient in pesto, basil is said to have a calming effect and aid digestion. Try basil tea after a rich meal or to relieve nausea.

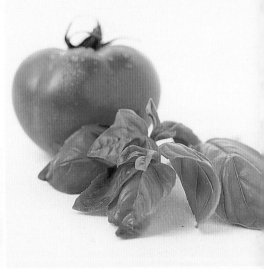

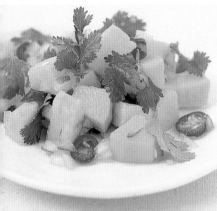

RECIPE Make a healthy fresh salsa from some ginger, pawpaw, chilli, red onion and coriander leaves. Serve with chicken or fish.

ROSEMARY May help to relieve indigestion. To add a subtle rosemary flavour to grilled meat, tie some rosemary sprigs together and use for basting.

PARSLEY High in vitamins A and C, it is delicious with egg and seafood dishes. Also a great sugarless breath freshener.

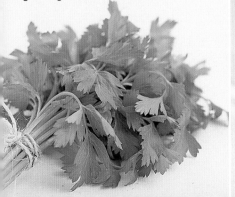

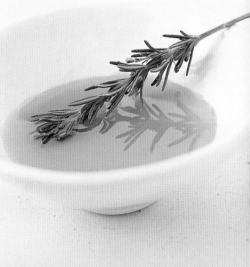

FOOD	CARB	FIBRE	FAT	ENERGY	
	g	g	g	kcal	kJ

ICE CREAM CONT.

FOOD	CARB	FIBRE	FAT	kcal	kJ
tub, chocolate, 100ml	9.5	0	5.5	92	385
tub, cookies & fudge, 100ml	14.5	0	16	215	905
tub, light & creamy vanilla, 100ml	15	0	1.5	77	325
tub, natural vanilla, 100ml	10	0	6	101	425
tub, original vanilla, 100ml	10	0	4.8	89	375
tub, original extra creamy vanilla, 100ml	10.5	0	5.5	99	415
tub, strawberries & cream, 100ml	22.5	0	10.5	198	830
tub, double choc, 100ml	21	0	13.5	218	915
tub, vanilla choc-chip, 100ml	N	0	6	106	445
tub, vanilla light, 100ml	12	0	3	83	350
vanilla, 100ml	21	0	10	187	785
viennetta style, chocolate, 100ml	13	0	9	133	559
viennetta style, toffee, 100ml	13	0	10	129	540
viennetta style, vanilla, 100ml	13	0	10	124	520

JAM

FOOD	CARB	FIBRE	FAT	kcal	kJ
apricot, reduced sugar, 1tbsp	4	+	0	17	70
average, all types, 1tbsp	17	+	0	67	280
berry, 1tbsp	17.5	+	0	68	285
fruits of the forest, reduced sugar, 1tbsp	4	+	0	17	70
marmalade, orange, 1tbsp	17	+	0	65	275
marmalade, reduced sugar, 1tbsp	4	+	0	17	70

JELLY

FOOD	CARB	FIBRE	FAT	kcal	kJ
jelly, low-sugar, prepared, 1 bowl, 270ml	0	0	0	24	100
jelly, prepared, 1 bowl, 280ml	45.5	0	0	188	790

JUICE (see INDIVIDUAL FRUITS)
KALE

FOOD	CARB	FIBRE	FAT	kcal	kJ
cooked, 65g	3.5	1.5	0.5	18	75
raw, 35g	3.5	1	0	18	75
KIWI FRUIT raw, peeled, 1 small, 75g	7.5	1.5	0	36	150
KOHL RABI peeled, boiled, 50g	2.5	1	0	18	75

LAMB

FOOD	CARB	FIBRE	FAT	kcal	kJ
chump chop, lean, grilled, 1, 55g	0	0	4.5	111	465
chump chop, untrimmed, grilled, 1, 65g	0	0	12	182	765
cutlet lean, grilled or baked, 1, 30g	0	0	4	70	295
cutlet, untrimmed, grilled or baked, 1, 40g	0	0	10.5	131	550
heart, baked, 70g	0	0	5.5	129	540
kidney, simmered, 150g	0	0	6.5	218	915
leg, lean, baked, 2 slices, 80g	0	0	5	158	665
leg, untrimmed, baked, 2 slices, 90g	0	0	10.5	201	845
liver, fried, 40g	0	0	5.5	96	405
loin chop, lean, grilled, 1, 35g	0	0	2.5	62	260
loin chop, untrimmed, grilled, 1, 50g	0	0	15.5	182	765
neck chop, lean, stewed, 1, 40g	0	0	5.5	101	425
neck chop, untrimmed, stewed, 1, 50g	0	0	14	176	740
shank, lean, cooked, 1, 130g	0	0	4.5	180	755
shank, untrimmed, cooked, 1, 100g	0	0	10.5	223	935
shoulder, lean, baked, 1 slice, 25g	0	0	2	46	195

LOW-FAT FROZEN FRUIT DESSERTS
Sometimes with less than 2g fat per serving, these desserts are guilt-free and come in a variety of flavours.

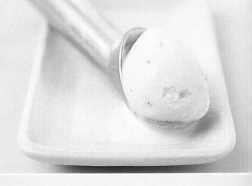

SORBET With no fat, this is a refreshing, but sweet, alternative to ice cream. Usually made with fruit, so it can be high in vitamin C.

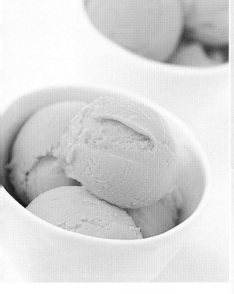

ICE CREAM As a general rule, the creamier the ice cream is, the higher the fat content. Ice cream is a good source of vitamins and calcium, but the milk or cream does add saturated fat. There are now many alternatives to ice cream in our supermarkets, including frozen fruit, tofu or yoghurt desserts – look out for the low-fat varieties.

GOURMET ICE CREAMS These often contain more fat than ordinary ice creams, but they are made with better-quality ingredients and sometimes contain real fruit.

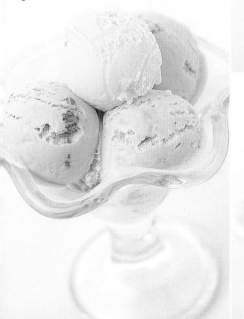

RECIPE For a tasty and quick dessert, layer a passionfruit, fat-free frozen dessert with sliced banana and a spoonful of low-fat honey vanilla yoghurt. Top with some chopped nuts.

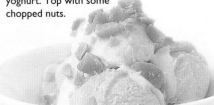

FOOD	CARB	FIBRE	FAT	ENERGY	
	g	g	g	kcal	kJ
LAMB CONT.					
shoulder, untrimmed, baked, 1 slice, 30g	0	0	6	87	365
trim, butterfly steak, grilled, 100g	0	0	4.5	125	525
trim, fillet, grilled, 100g	0	0	4	115	485.
trim, roast loin, baked, 100g	0	0	4	119	500
trim, schnitzel steak, grilled, 100g	0	0	3.5	111	465
strips, grilled, 100g	0	0	3.5	114	480
LASAGNE (see also PASTA)					
beef, commercial, 400g	62.8	2.8	24	572	2412
bolognaise, 400g	67.5	+	11.5	481	2020
lean beef lasagne, 400g	64	+	8.5	440	1850
LEEK sliced, boiled, 1 serving, 45g	1.2	0.8	0.3	9	39
LEMON					
curd, 1tbsp	10.5	0	3.5	76	320
juice, 100 ml	2.5	0	0	26	110
flavoured-spread, 1tbsp	13	0	1	60	250
raw, whole, 1, 65g	2.1	+	0	12	51
LENTILS					
burger, 1, 70g	15.5	2	1.5	213	895
dhal, 125g	14	2.5	9	177	745
dried, boiled, 200g	35	3.8	0.8	200	848
LETTUCE					
cos, 1 serving, 35g	0.6	0.3	0	6	25
iceberg, 35g	0.6	0.3	0	2	10
average, 35g	0.6	0.3	0	5	21
LIME					
juice, 1tbsp	2	0	0	6	25
raw, peeled, whole, 1, 45g	0.5	+	0	9	40
LINSEEDS (FLAXSEEDS) 1tbsp	4	+	4	58	245
LIQUORICE					
allsorts, 6, 56g	43	1	1.2	195	821
pieces, 5, 65g	42	1	1	181	759
LIVERWURST 60g	0.5	+	17.5	198	830
LOGANBERRIES raw, 100g	13	2.4	0.5	55	230
LOQUATS 6 medium, 78g	4	+	0	20	85
LOTUS ROOT					
canned, cooked, 100g	16	+	0	65	275
raw, peeled, 100g	17	+	0	74	310
LYCHEES					
canned in syrup, drained, 100g	17.7	0.5	0	68	290
raw, peeled, 100g	14.3	0.7	0.1	58	248
MACARONI					
cheese, homemade, 1 serving, 150g	20.4	0.8	16.2	267	1115
cheese, bought, 1 serving, 243g	49	1	15.5	405	1700
cheese, traditional, canned, 1 serving, 335g	71	1	21	557	2340
cheese & bacon, 1 serving, 293g	58	1	21	476	2000
cheesy fun shapes, 1 serving, 335g	71	1	21	557	2340
plain, boiled, 1 serving, 100g	18.5	0.9	0.5	86	365

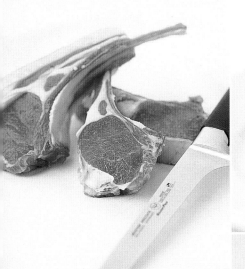

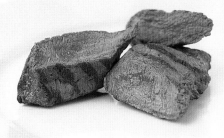

TRIM LAMB For a very lean cut of lamb, try eye of loin or backstrap. Avoid overcooking as lean cuts tend to dry out. Add to a stir-fry or try searing under the grill.

CUTTING FAT OFF LAMB When buying lamb, check how much fat you can see and whether it can be removed – a lamb cutlet that has been trimmed will have a lot less saturated fat. The leanest cuts are the leg and shank, the fattiest are the shoulder and rack.

DICED LAMB To make sure your diced lamb is lean, purchase lean cuts such as fillet or eye of loin and dice your own.

LAMB Although lamb was once considered to be a very fatty meat, changes in farming and breeding techniques have produced much leaner lamb that is widely available. Average, well-trimmed lamb can contain less than 8% fat, which is no more than many cuts of beef or pork. It's also worth trying out healthier methods of cooking, such as grilling, rather than just roasting.

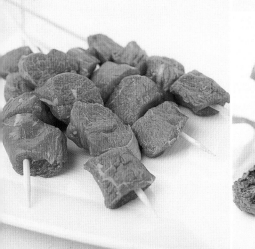

RECIPE For no-fuss, low-fat lamb, marinate trimmed lamb cutlets in tandoori paste, lemon juice and plain low-fat yoghurt overnight. Grill until tender.

FOOD	CARB g	FIBRE g	FAT g	ENERGY kcal	kJ
MANDARIN					
canned in juice, drained, 1 serving, 100g	7.7	0.3	0	32	135
peeled, whole, 1, 60g	5	1	0	24	100
MANGO					
canned in syrup, 200g	40.6	1.4	0	144	660
chutney, 1tbsp	8.5	0.5	0	34	145
green, 150g	25	3	0	58	245
ripe, raw, peeled, whole, 1, 150g	21.2	3.9	0.3	86	368
MARGARINE					
average, 1 portion, 11g	0.1	0	9	81	334
light, salt-reduced, 11g	0	0	4	36	150
lite, 1tsp, 5g	0	0	3	26	110
sunflower spread, 11g	0.1	0	7.3	67	274
dairy blend, extra-soft, 1tsp, 5g	0	0	3	26	110
blended, 1tsp, 5g	0	0	3.5	31	130
butter type, 1tsp, 5g	0	0	4	36	150
high polyunsaturated spread, 1tsp	0	0	4	33	140
olive oil, type, 1tsp, 5g	0	0	4	33	140
sunflower spread, fat-reduced, 1 tsp, 5g	0	0	2.5	21	90
MARROW					
peeled, boiled, 100g	4	0.5	0	19	80
raw, peeled, 100g	3.5	0.5	0	17	70
MARZIPAN 20g	11	0.6	3.5	80	335
MATZO					
meal, 50g	40	+	0	171	720
plain cracker, 30g	25	1	0.5	118	495
MAYONNAISE					
97% fat free, 1tbsp	9	0	20	45	190
cholesterol free, 1tbsp	7.5	0	3.5	63	265
sunflower type, 1tbsp	7.5	0	7.5	107	450
light, 1tbsp	8	0	7	63	265
olive oil type, 1tbsp	5	0	8.5	97	410
premium type, 1tbsp	7	0	3	58	245
traditional, 1tbsp	3	0	21.5	201	845
reduced calorie, 1tbsp	7	0	3	55	230
MEAT SUBSTITUTES					
micro protein, 100g	2	4.8	3.5	86	360
vegetarian mince, 100g	22	1.4	2.5	304	1280
MELON					
casaba, raw, peeled, 100g	6	0.4	0	32	135
honeydew, raw, peeled, 160g	10.5	0.6	0.5	50	210
rock, raw, peeled, 250g	12	1	0	55	230
water, raw, peeled, 100g	5	0.2	0	23	95
MERINGUE 25g	22.5	0	0	92	385
MILK					
buttermilk, cultured, dairy, 1 carton, 250ml	4	0	5.5	132	555
calcium enriched, 1 cup, 250ml	12.5	0	2.5	119	500

MILK Is an excellent source of calcium and protein and also contains vitamins and minerals. It is an essential part of many people's diet, and is particularly important for infants and young children.

WHOLE MILK Relatively high in saturated fat, whole milk does contain more vitamin A and D than skimmed varieties.

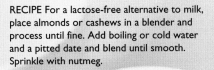

CALCIUM It is recommended that adults consume 700mg calcium every day, in order to maintain healthy bones. This is about the amount available in a pint of milk (any variety).

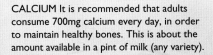

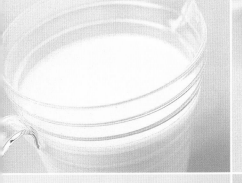

RECIPE For a lactose-free alternative to milk, place almonds or cashews in a blender and process until fine. Add boiling or cold water and a pitted date and blend until smooth. Sprinkle with nutmeg.

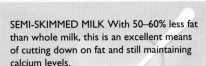

SKIMMED MILK Although this lacks the fat-soluble vitamins A and D, skimmed milk has the same amount of calcium as other varieties.

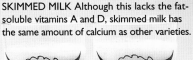

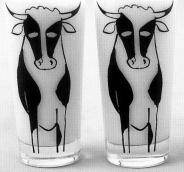

SEMI-SKIMMED MILK With 50–60% less fat than whole milk, this is an excellent means of cutting down on fat and still maintaining calcium levels.

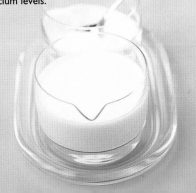

FOOD	CARB	FIBRE	FAT	ENERGY	
	g	g	g	kcal	kJ
MILK CONT.					
condensed, sweetened, 1 tin, 250ml	180	0	30	1060	4455
condensed, sweetened, skim, 250ml	199	0	1	901	3785
cultured, reduced-fat, 250ml	12	0	5	134	565
cultured, skim, 250ml	14.5	0	0.5	108	455
evaporated, reduced-fat, canned, 250ml	28.5	0	5.5	241	1015
evaporated, skim, canned, 250ml	28.5	0	1	200	840
evaporated, whole-fat, canned, 250ml	27	0	21.5	373	1565
fat-reduced, protein-increased, 250ml	14	0	3.5	126	530
flavoured, chocolate, 250ml	23	0	9.5	204	855
flavoured, chocolate, reduced-fat, 1 cup, 250ml	21.5	0	4.5	156	655
flavoured, malt & honey, 250ml	27	0	2.5	170	715
flavoured, strawberry, 250ml	23	0	9	201	845
flavoured, strawberry, reduced-fat, 250ml	24	0	4	158	665
full-cream, 250ml	12	0	10	167	700
goat's, 1 cup, 250ml	9.5	0	6.5	127	535
lite, 250ml	14.5	0	3.5	133	558
low-fat, high-calcium, 250ml	17	0	0.5	120	505
milkshake, 275ml	47	0	12	349	1465
milkshake, thick, 300ml	60	0	10	355	1490
powder, malted, 1tbsp	5.5	0	0.5	32	135
powdered, full-cream, 1tbsp	3	0	2	39	165
powdered, skim, 1tbsp	4	0	0	29	120
rice, 250ml	N	0	2.5	157	660
sheep's, 250ml	13.5	0	17.5	268	1125
skimmed, 250ml	12.5	0	0.5	88	370
soya, natural, 250ml	18.5	+	7	158	665
soya, low-fat, 250ml	12	N	1.8	91	382
soya, lite, 250ml	15	N	1.5	107	450
soya, flavoured, banana, 250ml	23	+	2	138	580
soya, flavoured, chocolate hazelnut, 250ml	18.5	5	7	158	665
MILLET					
cooked, 174g	41	+	1.5	206	865
MISO (SOYA BEAN PASTE) 1tbsp	6	+	1	40	170
MIXED PEEL 100g	59	4.8	1	231	984
MIXED VEGETABLES					
frozen, boiled, 1 serving 100g	6.6	+	0.5	42	180
MOLASSES 1tbsp	14	0	0	54	225
MUESLI (see CEREAL)					
MUESLI BAR (see also CEREAL BAR)					
apricot & coconut, 1 bar, 31g	19.5	N	7.5	149	625
apricot & fibre, yoghurt-coated bar,					
1 bar, 50g	28	+	9.5	202	850
brown rice, macadamia & ginger, 1 bar, 50g	26	+	14	234	985
chewy fruit, 1 bar, 31g	21	1	5	131	550
crunchy fruit, 1 bar, 31g	17.5	1.2	7	146	615
crunchy original, yoghurt, 1 bar, 31g	22	+	4	126	530
fruit, apricot, 1 bar, 32g	22.5	+	4.5	137	575

BUTTERMILK A low-fat alternative to milk, buttermilk has a slightly sour taste and can be used in cooking to replace whole milk.

SOYA MILK As it is not a natural source of calcium, many varieties have calcium added. However, they may also be sweetened so avoid frequent consumption.

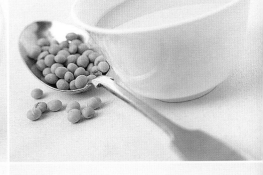

EVAPORATED MILK This is milk that has had much of its water evaporated. Look for low-fat varieties, which can replace cream in cooking.

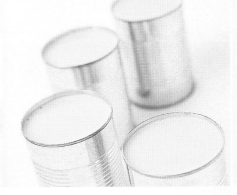

MILK Although dairy products are an important part of a healthy diet, they are also relatively high in saturated fat and should be consumed in moderation. However, simply cutting back on dairy products may result in a lower calcium intake, so instead try replacing them with lower fat alternatives, which will not affect calcium levels.

RICE MILK A high-carbohydrate drink, rice milk is a good option for those who are lactose-intolerant. It is sweeter than soy milk.

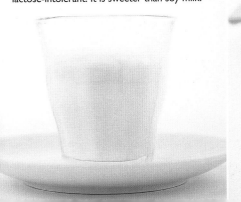

MILK POWDER This loses little of the nutritional value associated with normal milk.

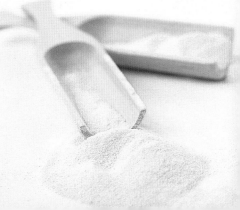

FOOD	CARB	FIBRE	FAT	ENERGY	
	g	g	g	kcal	kJ
MUESLI BAR CONT.					
nut crumble, 1 bar, 31g	20	+	6	143	600
nut & muesli, carob-coated, 1 bar, 50g	28	+	11	218	915
peach & pear, 100% fruit, 1 bar, 25g	15	N	8.6	131	550
yoghurt, apricot, 1 bar, 31g	20.5	+	5.5	138	580
yoghurt tops, fruit salad, 1 bar, 31g	21.5	+	5	136	570
MUFFIN					
1 medium, plain, 60g	29	1.5	8	169	710
1 large, 100g	48	2	13	279	1170
1 extra large, 150g	72	3	19.5	418	1755
blueberry, 1, 150g	56	+	13	352	1480
bran, 1, 190g	67	15	27.5	550	2310
calorie-reduced, 1, 152g	47.5	+	18	370	1555
high-fibre, 1, 63g	27.5	+	2	152	640
fruit, 1, 60g	27	+	1.5	151	635
soya & linseed, 1, 67g	N	++	6.5	180	755
spicy fruit topped, 1, 67g	30	+	2	168	705
white, bread type, 1, 67g	28.5	2	1	151	635
wholemeal, bread type, 1, 67g	N	+	2	156	655
low-fat, 1, 152g	57.5	+	2.5	283	1190
mixed berry, 1, 60g	38	+	5	207	870
muffin mix, apple & sultana, prepared, 1, 60g	33	+	7	202	850
muffin mix, blueberry & apricot, prepared, 1, 60g	32	+	6.7	202	850
muffin mix, choc-chip, prepared, 1, 60g	32	N	7	213	895
MULBERRIES					
raw, 100g	4.5	++	0	29	120
MUSHROOMS					
button, raw, 100g	1.5	1.1	0.5	24	100
canned, 100g	1.5	1.3	0.5	15	65
canned in butter sauce, 100g	3.5	1	1	27	115
champignon, canned, 100g	1	1	0	13	55
chinese, dried & rehydrated, 25g	4	N	0	14	60
enoki, raw, 100g	7	N	0.5	35	145
oyster, raw, 100g	6	+	0.5	37	155
shiitake, dried, 4, 15g	11	+	0	44	185
straw, canned, drained, 100g	4.5	+	0.5	32	135
swiss brown, 100g	N	+	0	23	95
MUSTARD					
American, 1tbsp	1	0	0	15	65
English, 1tbsp	1	0	0	15	65
French, 1tbsp	1	0	0	15	65
powder, wholegrain, 1tsp, 5g	0.5	1	1	18	75
seeded, 1tbsp	1	+	0	15	65
NASHI PEAR					
raw, unpeeled, 1, 130g	9.2	2	0	38	158
NECTARINE					
raw, unpeeled, 1, 75g	6.75	1	0	30	126

CAROB-COATED BARS An alternative to chocolate, carob has the same amount of fat but is free of caffeine.

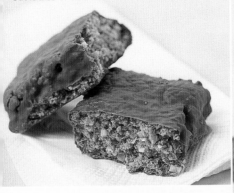

BREAKFAST BARS A good breakfast is a great way to start the day but if you don't have time, bars can be a convenient alternative to cereal.

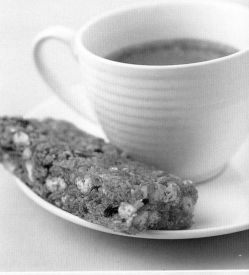

MUESLI & CEREAL BARS Often

eaten as a quick snack, muesli bars can be a good source of dietary fibre and may be a healthier snack option than a packet of crisps or a chocolate bar. However, they are not always as healthy as they seem and can contain up to 17g of fat and lots of sugar per bar. Check the label carefully.

MUESLI BARS Some varieties are high in sugar and provide a great energy boost when eaten before or after exercise. If you are not that active, they may provide more energy than you need.

YOGHURT-COATED BARS Handy for a picnic or lunch box, some contain real fruit. Check the fat content on the label.

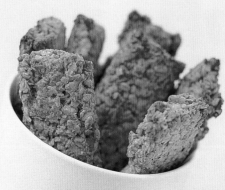

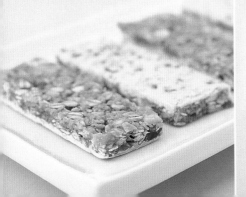

FOOD	CARB	FIBRE	FAT	ENERGY	
	g	g	g	kcal	kJ
NOODLES					
egg, boiled, 1 portion, 100g	13	0.6	0.5	62	264
instant, boiled, 1 portion, 100g	N	+	5	367	1540
rice, boiled, 1 portion, 100g	21.5	0.5	0.5	99	415
rice, fried, 1 portion, 150g	16.8	0.8	17.2	230	964
rice, vermicelli, boiled, 30g	N	+	0.5	110	460
buckwheat, boiled, 100g	21.5	+	0	99	415
quick-cook noodles, all flavours, 1 packet, 85g	54	+	16	390	1640
noodles, rice, dry, 100g	81.5	+	0.1	360	1506
wheat, fried, 80g	50	+	17	374	1570
wheat, steamed, 80g	60	+	2	283	1190
NUTMEAT					
canned, 100g	6	+	8.5	195	820
NUTS					
almond, blanched, 85g	5.8	6.3	47.5	520	2185
almond, chocolate-coated, 75g	49.5	4.5	33.5	517	2170
almond, raw, 4	0.5	1.5	8	87	365
almond, raw & unpeeled, 85g	2	2.3	17.5	195	817
almond, smoked, 30g	1.5	N	15	194	815
almond, sugar-coated, 30g	N	N	12	130	545
brazil, raw, 80g	2.5	3.4	54.5	546	2291
cashew, raw, 75g	13.6	2.4	36	430	1805
cashew, roasted, 75g	14	2.4	38	458	1925
chestnut, raw, 72g	26	3	2	122	514
hazelnut, raw, 70g	4.2	4.5	44.4	455	1911
macadamia, salted, 73g	3.5	3.8	56.6	546	2293
mixed, 78g	6	4.7	42	473	1988
mixed nuts & raisins, 100g	31.5	4.5	34	481	2004
peanut, raw, 78g	9.75	4.8	35.9	440	1848
peanut, roasted, 78g	8	5	38.8	459	1930
pecan, raw, 55g	3.2	2.6	38.5	379	1592
pinenut, raw, 1 tbsp, 15g	0.6	0.3	10.2	103	433
pistachio, raw, 63g	5	3.8	35	379	1590
walnut chopped, raw, 55g	1.8	2	38	378	1589
OATMEAL 40g	29	2.7	3.5	160	674
OIL					
blended, 1tbsp	0	0	20	176	740
cod liver, 1tbsp	0	0	20	176	740
olive oil, 1tbsp	0	0	19	167	703
OKRA					
boiled, 6 pods, 65g	1	2.3	0	13	55
OLIVES					
black, 6 medium, 40g	N	N	7	39	165
green, 6 medium, 50g	Tr	1.5	5.5	56	211
stuffed, 5 olives, 20g	0.5	1.5	1.5	18	75
ONION					
brown, raw, peeled, 1 medium, 100g	4.5	1.4	0	24	100
pickled, drained, 2, 36g	4.5	0.4	0	21	90

RECIPE To make your own basil oil, simply heat some extra virgin olive oil, then add fresh herbs and cool. Process, then strain and use immediately.

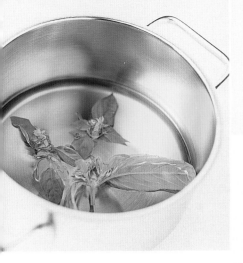

OIL All oils contain roughly the same amount of fat, but the important issue is the type of fat. Palm and coconut oils, often used for frying, are high in saturated fat and should be avoided, while the other oils have more monounsaturated and polyunsaturated fats, both of which have health benefits.

MONOUNSATURATED OILS These oils, such as olive, canola or peanut, are thought to lower blood cholesterol when they replace saturated fat in the diet.

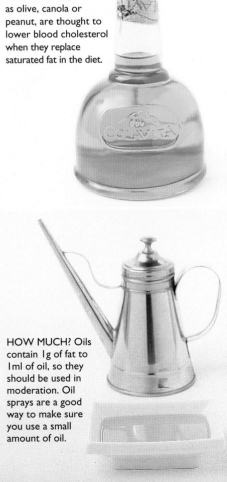

POLYUNSATURATED OILS These oils, such as sunflower or corn oil, contain essential fatty acids that the body cannot produce itself. They may also lower blood cholesterol when they replace saturated fats in the diet.

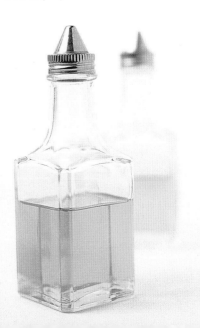

HOW MUCH? Oils contain 1g of fat to 1ml of oil, so they should be used in moderation. Oil sprays are a good way to make sure you use a small amount of oil.

FOOD	CARB g	FIBRE g	FAT g	ENERGY kcal	ENERGY kJ
ONION CONT.					
red, raw, peeled, I small, 100g	4.5	1.4	0	25	105
spring, raw, whole, 1, 14g	0.5	0.2	0	3	14
white, raw, peeled, I medium, 100g	4.5	1.4	0	26	110
ORANGE					
all varieties, raw, peeled, 120g	10.2	2	0	44	186
juice, freshly squeezed, 100ml	8.1	0.1	0	33	140
juice, commercial, unsweetened, 100ml	8.8	0.1	0	36	153
PANCAKE					
average, homemade, 1, 16 cm, 50g	14	0.5	1	75	315
PAPADUM					
fried, 3 small, 10g	3.9	N	1.7	37	155
grilled or microwaved, 3 small	N	N	0	17	70
PAPAYA (PAWPAW)					
raw, peeled, 100g	8.8	2.2	0	36	153
canned in juice,100g	17	0.7	0	65	275
PARSNIP raw, peeled, boiled, 100g	12.9	4.7	1.2	66	278
PASSIONFRUIT I average, 40g	2.5	1.5	0	19	80
PASTA (see also LASAGNE AND SPAGHETTI)					
egg, cooked, I serving, 200g	51	2	1	261	1095.
plain, all shapes, cooked, I serving, 180g	44.5	1.8	0.5	213	895
ravioli, cheese & spinach, cooked, I serving, 265g	88	+	16.5	640	2690
ravioli, meat, cooked, I serving, 265g	82.5	+	17.5	602	2530
spinach, cooked, I serving, 200g	54.5	+	1	258	1085
tomato & herb fettucine, cooked, 200g	39	+	1.5	186	780
tortellini, cheese & spinach, cooked, I serving, 265g	88	+	16.5	640	2690
tortellini, meat, I serving	N	N	5	379	1590
wholemeal, cooked, I serving, 180g	42	6.3	1.6	203	854
PASTA SAUCE					
carbonara, jar, I serving, 125g	21.5	+	6.5	158	665
creamy mushroom, I serving, 280g	25	+	0.5	119	500
spicy tomato, I serving, 125g	20.5	+	5	140	589
tomato, bottled, I serving, 280g	26.5	+	2	134	565
PASTRY					
choux, cooked, 30g	9	0.4	7	108	454
filo, 2 sheets	15	N	0.5	77	325
flaky, average portion, cooked, 50g	23	0.9	20.3	280	1176
hot-water, 50g	27	N	10	213	895
puff, I sheet, 170g	63	N	42.3	671	2820
shortcrust, cooked, 100g	54.2	2.2	32.3	521	2174
strudel, 50g	23	N	20	267	1120
suet crust, 50g	27	N	10	213	895
wholemeal, cooked, 100g	44.6	6.3	32.9	499	2080
PATE					
chicken liver, 1 tbsp	N	0	2.5	27	112
country, 1 tbsp	0.5	0.5	5	59	250
PAVLOVA					
pavlova shell mix, prepared, I serving, 60g	4	0	0	173	725

RECIPE For a quick and healthy pasta sauce, cook a chopped onion and garlic clove in a non-stick pan until soft. Add a little red or white wine and some fresh chopped tomatoes and toss together until heated through. Sprinkle with slivers of Parmesan.

CREAMY SAUCES You can make low-fat versions of cream sauces like Alfredo and Carbonara using stock, low-fat milk and some cornflour to thicken.

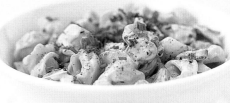

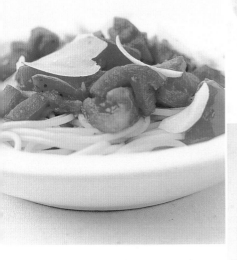

PASTA & PASTA SAUCE

High in starchy carbohydrates and low in fat, pasta is a healthy way to fill up. However, it's the pasta sauce that can pile on the fat and calories. Always serve plenty of pasta with only a relatively small amount of topping, and opt for a homemade tomato sauce, rather than high-fat creamy or cheesy sauces.

WHOLEMEAL PASTA With over twice the dietary fibre of plain pasta, wholemeal is particularly good in pasta bakes and salads.

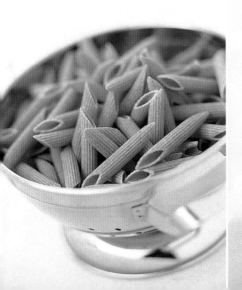

PLAIN PASTA Though the flour used to make plain pasta has had the wheatgerm and bran removed, it still contains plenty of fibre and starch.

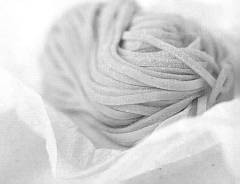

FOOD	CARB g	FIBRE g	FAT g	ENERGY kcal	kJ
PAVLOVA CONT.					
shell, with cream & passion fruit, I serving	N	+	11	315	1325
PAWPAW whole, raw, 100g	7	2	0	30	125
PEACH					
canned in jelly, snack pack	N	N	0	95	400
canned in juice, drained, 140g	12.5	1.2	0	56	235
canned in syrup, 250g	14	2.2	0	61	255
dried, 25g	13	1.8	0	61	255
raw, I medium, 140g	9	2	0	44	185
stewed, with sugar, 100g	25.5	2.9	0.5	106	445
stewed, without sugar, 100g	21.5	3	0.5	92	385
PEAR					
canned, snack pack 140g	N	2	0	82	345
canned in pear juice, drained, 250g	25.5	3.5	0	106	445
canned in syrup, drained, 250g	37	2.75	0	148	620
canned in water, drained, 250g	16	3.5	0	64	270
dried, 2, 87g	60.5	7.2	0.5	227	955
juice, canned, 200ml	27.5	0	0	112	470
raw, unpeeled, 185g	18.5	4	0	74	311
PEAS					
green, cooked, I serving, 165g	10.5	7.4	0.5	80	335
peas, raw, 170g	10	8	I	98	410
split, dried, cooked, I serving, 180g	12	4.9	I	104	435
sugar snap, 170g	10	2.2	I	98	410
PHEASANT raw, meat only, 125g	0	0	4.5	165	695
PIGEON breast, lean, roasted, 125g	0	0	14.5	263	1105
PINEAPPLE					
canned in juice, drained, I bowl, 250ml	25.5	1.25	0	112	470
canned in syrup, drained, I slice, 40g	8	0.3	0	33	140
juice, unsweetened, canned, 250ml	27	0	0	111	465
raw, peeled, I slice, 110g	9	1.3	0	42	175
PIE meat, average,					
all types, 1, 190g	34	0.8	26	429	1800
PIZZA (see FAST FOOD)					
PLUM					
canned in syrup, drained, I serving, 225g	35	1.8	0.3	132	557
raw, 100g	8.8	1.6	0	36	155
stewed, without sugar, I serving, 250g	17	4	0	85	357
POLENTA dry, 60g	41	+	I	198	830.
POMEGRANATE raw, peeled, 100g	11.8	3.4	0.2	51	218
POPCORN					
caramel-coated, 100g	77.6	N	20	480	2018
plain, commercial, 2 scoops, 16g	8.5	N	4	75	315
PORK					
bacon, breakfast rasher, grilled, 1, 34g	0	0	1.5	48	200
barbecued, Chinese-style, 100g	3.5	N	15	233	980
belly, rasher, untrimmed, grilled, 100g	0	0	22	298	1250
crackling, 30g	0	0	9	142	610

PORK

Thought of as a fatty meat, pork is now bred to be leaner. In fact, lean cuts of pork often have less fat than beef, lamb and chicken. However, other pork products, such as salami, sausages, spare ribs and bacon, have a much higher fat content in general, and are also quite high in saturated fat.

BACON The fat content of bacon can be reduced by up to 50%, simply by trimming off all visible fat and grilling rather than frying.

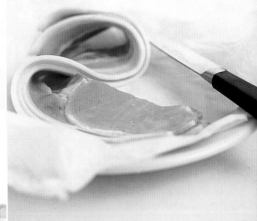

RECIPE To cook lean pork, fry lean steaks in a non-stick pan until brown and tender. Remove, then add some sliced apple, wholegrain mustard and apple cider to the pan. Simmer until the apples are soft, add the steaks and reheat.

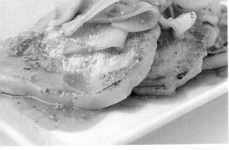

FILLET The leanest cut of pork, this is an excellent substitute for beef or lamb in stir-fries. Alternatively, cut the fillet into slices and grill or barbecue.

LEAN STEAKS Lean pork steaks are ideal for grilling or pan-frying with little or no added fat. Always remove visible fat before cooking.

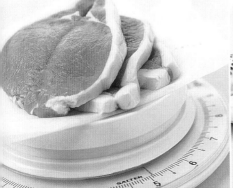

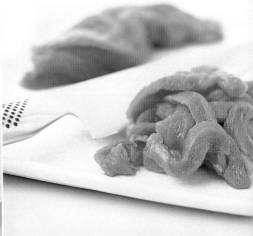

FOOD	CARB	FIBRE	FAT	ENERGY	
	g	g	g	kcal	kJ
PORK CONT.					
fillet lean, baked, 1, 100g	0	0	5	169	710
forequarter chop, lean, grilled, 1, 95g	0	0	7.5	171	720
forequarter chop, untrimmed, grilled, 1, 100g	0	0	28.5	343	1440
leg roast, lean, 2 slices, 95g	0	0	4	163	685
leg roast with fat, 2 slices, 100g	0	0	26.5	338	1420
leg, lean, grilled, 1, 100g	0	0	3.5	156	655
leg, untrimmed, grilled, 1, 100g	0	0	6	171	720
loin chop, lean, grilled. 1, 100g	0	0	5.5	174	730
loin chop, untrimmed, grilled, 1, 100g	0	0	30	362	1520
medallion steak, lean, grilled, 1 small, 100g	0	0	5.5	187	785
medallion steak, untrimmed, grilled,					
1 small, 100g	0	0	22.5	307	1290
mince, 100g	0	0	30	75	315
pie, 1, 180g	46.5	1.8	53.5	763	3205
ribs, spare, 100g	0	0	10	114	480
steak, lean, grilled, 100g	0	0	4.5	161	675
steak untrimmed, grilled, 100g	0	0	17.5	259	1090
POTATO					
baked, jacket, no oil, 1 medium, 150g	21.5	2	1	109	460
boiled, peeled, 1 medium, 150g	19.5	1.5	0.5	96	405
boiled, unpeeled, 1 medium, 150g	20	2	0	98	410
chips, oven-cook, frozen, cooked, 100g	25	2	3	131	550
fries (thin-cut), medium serving	43	1	18	338	1420
oven-fried, 100g	29	6	13	245	1030
hash brown, 1 average, 55g	15	1	12	171	720
mashed with milk & butter, 1 serving, 120g	N	2.5	1	77	325
mashed with skim milk, 120g	N	2.5	0	71	300
new, peeled, boiled, 3, 165g	21	3	0	103	435
roast, no skin, 150g	26	2.5	4	159	670
roast, with skin. 150g	25	2	4	159	670
steamed, new, peeled, 165g	20	3	0	102	430
wedges, crunchy, 100g	26	4.5	6	165	695
POTATO CRISPS					
(see CORN CHIPS AND SNACK FOOD)					
PRICKLY PEAR raw, peeled, 86g	7.5	N	0	34	145
PRUNES					
dried, 5, 38g	16.5	2.2	0	70	295
juice, 250ml	44.5	Tr	0	181	760.
stewed, with sugar, 150g	29.5	4.6	0	119	500
stewed, without sugar, 150g	18.5	4.8	0	78	330
PUMPKIN					
peeled, boiled, 85g	6	1	0.5	36	150
pie, 1 slice, 109g	29.5	3	10.5	229	960
roasted in oil with 1/2tbsp oil, 85g	8	1.5	8	125	525
seeds, dry roasted, 1tbsp	4.5	1	11.5	134	565
PURSLANE					
boiled, 1 cup, 115g	4	N	0	20	85

WEDGES For a healthy alternative to chips, lightly spray potato wedges with oil and bake in a 200°C (400°F/Gas 6) oven for 40 minutes until golden.

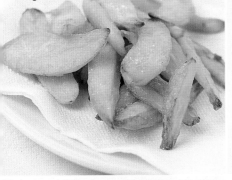

POTATO High in carbohydrate, potassium and vitamin C, potatoes are a great staple food – it's just the way they're cooked, and their affinity with butter and salt, that can make them unhealthy. Baking is a healthy way to cook potatoes. Boiled potatoes are also low in fat, but some of the vitamin C may be lost in the cooking water.

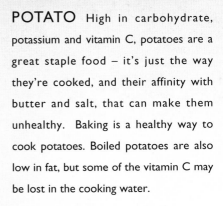

MASH You can make delicious mashed potatoes without too much butter. Use skimmed milk or stock, or try adding a little olive oil instead of the butter.

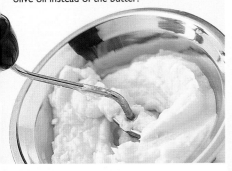

STEAMING A great way to cook potatoes and retain more vitamin C than boiling. Add some fresh herbs rather than lots of butter and salt.

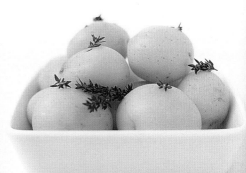

NEW POTATOES There are many potato varieties now available. Make a delicious salad with new potatoes and fresh herbs.

FRIES Fried potatoes are all fatty, but the thicker the chip, the less fat is absorbed during cooking. If you love fries, choose wedges.

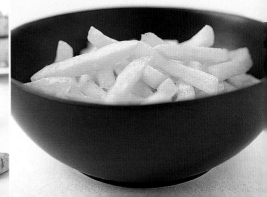

FOOD	CARB g	FIBRE g	FAT g	ENERGY kcal	ENERGY kJ
QUAIL					
roasted, with skin, 180g	0	0	6	180	755
roasted, without skin, 125g	0	0	20	349	1465
QUICHE					
cheese & egg, average homemade,					
slice, 125g	21.5	1	27.5	390	1640
lorraine, average, 100g	18	N	22	293	1230
mushroom, average homemade, 1 slice, 125g	23	1.5	24.5	352	1480
vegetable, average, 100g	20	N	18	259	1090
QUINCE					
raw, 100g	11	++	0	48	200
stewed, with added sugar, 100g	21	+	0	83	350
RABBIT meat only, baked, 100g	0	0	5.5	169	710
RADISH					
red, raw, 3, 45g	1	0.5	0	0.6	2.5
white, raw, peeled, sliced, 90g	2.5	1.5	0.5	15	65
RAISINS 100g	69.3	2	0.4	272	1159
RASPBERRIES					
canned in syrup, drained, 100g	22.5	1.5	0	88	374
raw, 65g	3	1.6	0.2	16	71
REDCURRANTS raw, 100g	14	3.4	0	56	235
RELISH					
corn, 1tbsp	4.5	0.2	0	20	85
mustard, 1tbsp	4.5	N	0	20	85
tomato, 1tbsp	4.5	0.2	0	19	80
RHUBARB					
raw, 100g	0.8	1.4	0	7	32
stewed with sugar, 125g	14.5	1.5	0	60	252
RICE					
average, cooked, 100g	33.4	0.1	1.1	157	660
basmati, cooked, 1 serving	42	+	0.3	177	742
brown, cooked, 1 serving, 180g	57	1.5	2	270	1135
extra-long grain, cooked, 70g	54.5	0.5	0.5	232	973
fragrant, cooked, 100g	34.6	0.5	0.4	155	651
fried, 190g	56	1.1	16	413	1735
long grain, cooked, 100g	34.6	+	0.4	155	651
white, cooked, 1 serving, 190g	53	0.2	0.5	237	995
wild, cooked, 1 serving, 164g	35	+	N	165	695
RICE CAKES					
corn & buckwheat, 1, 12g	10	+	0	49	205
corn cakes, natural, 2, 10g	9	+	0	36	150
natural brown, 2, 10g	8	+	0.5	14	60
rice & rye, 2, 10g	8	+	0.5	39	165
SAFFRON 1tbsp	1.5	0	0	6	25
SALADS					
bean salad, commercial, 1 serving, 210g	27	6.3	18	309	1298
coleslaw, commercial, 1 carton, 200g	8.4	2.8	52.8	516	1872
potato salad, 1 carton, 180g	20.5	1.4	47	517	1913

RICE

RICE The main staple of half the people in the world and an excellent source of energy, rice makes the perfect accompaniment to any meal as it gives a feeling of fullness without adding fat. When mixed with legumes, rice forms a complete protein, which is particularly important for vegetarians. It is also a gluten-free alternative to bread.

WHITE RICE The bran layer is removed during processing, leaving white rice lower in thiamin than wholegrain rice.

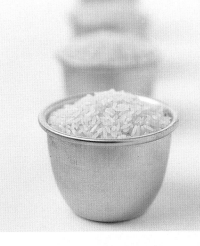

RECIPE Next time you make a soup, add some cooked rice to it. It will help to thicken it and raise carbohydrate levels.

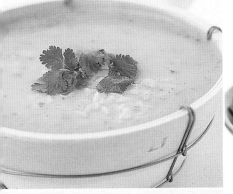

WILD RICE Not a true rice, but a grass native to North America. It can be blended with brown or white rice to add a delicious nutty flavour to dishes.

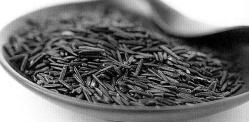

RICE PREFERENCES Although white varieties of rice may contain less fibre than wholegrain types, they are still nutritious and many people prefer the less distinctive flavour.

WHOLEGRAIN RICE This contains more fibre than white varieties. Although it can take longer to cook, it has a delicious, nutty flavour.

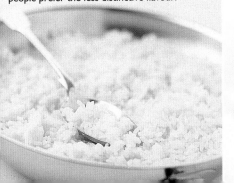

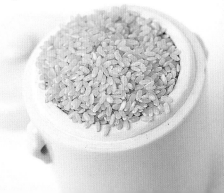

FOOD	CARB	FIBRE	FAT	ENERGY	
	g	g	g	kcal	kJ
SALAMI					
average, all varieties, 50g	0.5	0	19	214	900
Danish, 4 slices, 20g	0.5	N	8	88	370
pepperoni, 4 slices, 20g	0.5	0	7	80	335
SAUCES					
mayonnaise, 1tbsp	0.1	0	13	118	495
apricot chicken, 1 serving, 118g	15	0	1	69	290
apricot chicken, jar, 1 serving, 115g	16	0	10.5	67	280
barbecue, 1 tbsp	10	0	0	40	170
beef & black bean, 115g	11	0	1.5	58	245
bolognaise, 160g	3.5	N	14	192	805
butterscotch, 45g	15	0	17	214	900
chilli, 20g	10.5	0	0	9	40
country French chicken, 118g	5	0	11.5	126	530
creamy lemon chicken, 118g	15	0	0.7	69	290
creamy mushroom, 1 serving, 120g	6.5	0	1.5	133	560
golden honey mustard, 118g	12	0	13	170	715
gravy, commercial, 60g	5.5	0	5.5	81	340
gravy, made from powder, prepared, 60g	2.5	0	0	14	60
herbed chicken & wine, 1 serving, 115g	7.5	0	6.5	14	60
honey & sesame, 1 serving, 120g	23	0	1	108	455
honey, sesame & garlic, 1 serving, 115g	23	0	0.5	85	400
Hungarian goulash, 1 serving, 125g	7.5	0	3.5	105	440
Malaysian satay, 1tbsp	5	+	5	67	280
mild Indian, 1 serving, 115g	8	0	7	93	390
mint homemade, 1 tbsp	0	0	0	9	40
mornay, bought, 1 serving, 120g	5	0	14	161	675
onion, made from powdered mix, prepared, 125g	8.5	0	7	110	460
oyster, 1 tbsp	5	0	0	29	120
packet, average all types, 1 serving, 125g	10	0	20	263	1105
pesto, 1 tbsp	9	+	5	90	380
soya, 1 tbsp	0.5	0	0	9	40
spicy plum, 1 serving, 115g	21	N	0.5	86	360
sweet & sour, 1 serving, 115g	30.5	N	0	120	505
sweet & sour, lite, 1 serving, 115g	20.5	N	0	80	335
sweet Thai chilli, 115g	52.5	N	0.5	204	855
toffee, 1, 20g	15	0	2	80	335
tomato, 1tbsp	5.5	+	0	23	95
white, homemade, 1tbsp	2.5	+	5	27	115
worcestershire, 1tbsp	4	0	0	17	70
SAUSAGE					
beef, fried, homemade, 1, 50g	2	0.3	9	117	490
beef, grilled, homemade, 1, 50g	3	0.3	9	127	535
Bierschinken, 1, 30g	0	0	5	309	1300
black pudding, grilled, 1, 90g	6.5	+	21	281	1180
bratwurst, 100g	0	0	30	362	1520
cabanossi, 1, 30g	0	N	10	109	460
chicken, thin, 2, 50g	0	0	6	89	375

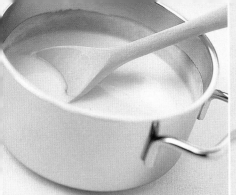

WHITE SAUCE For a low-fat alternative to this creamy sauce, use skimmed milk and replace the flour and butter with cornflour.

TOMATO SAUCE
High in sugar and sodium, but lower in fat than mayonnaise-based sauces.

SAUCES If you are using a small quantity of a sauce like tomato ketchup, you don't need to worry too much about its nutritional value. However, some sauces, especially cheesy or creamy sauces, can be high in fat. Ready-made commercial sauces tend also to be high in salt. Where possible, make your own, healthy varieties.

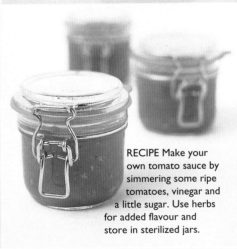

RECIPE Make your own tomato sauce by simmering some ripe tomatoes, vinegar and a little sugar. Use herbs for added flavour and store in sterilized jars.

COOK-IN SAUCES Can be high in fat and additives, so check the labels. Next time you make a tomato sauce, freeze half so you can add to meat or pasta for an instant dinner.

MINT SAUCE Make your own low-calorie version by mixing a handful of chopped mint leaves with a teaspoon of sugar, boiling water, and 3–4 tablespoons of white wine vinegar.

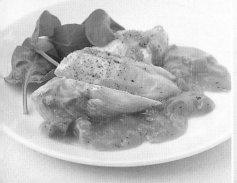

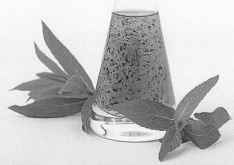

FOOD	CARB	FIBRE	FAT	ENERGY	
	g	g	g	kcal	kJ
SAUCES CONT.					
chicken, thin, low-fat, 2, 40g	0	0	3	70	295
chipolates (skinless), 2, 25g	0	0	5	55	230
Italian, cooked, 100g	0	0	30	362	1520
Chinese sausage, 100g	3	0	40	429	1800
low-fat, 1, 50g	0	0	5	75	315
pork, thick, grilled, 2, 150g	9	1	33	425	1785
pork, thin, grilled, 2, 100g	6	0.7	21.5	283	1190
Schinkenwurst, 30g	0	0	15	154	645
vegetarian, 1, 60g	4	1	4	98	410
SCONE					
fruit, 1, 50g	20	+	3	118	495
plain, average, 1, 50g	23	1	5	154	645
SEAFOOD					
baked, 85g	0	0	1	95	400
anchovies, canned in oil, drained, 5, 18g	0	0	1.5	33	140
bass, 100g	0	0	1	93	390
blackfish, 100g	0	0	2	93	390
blue grenadier, 100g	0	0	2	93	390
blue threadfin, 100g	0	0	2	93	390
boarfish, 100g	0	0	2	93	390
bream, steamed, 1 fillet, 149g	0	0	8	206	865
calamari tubes, raw, 100g	0	0	0	69	290
calamari tubes, fried, 100g	12	N	17.5	276	1160
caviar, black, 1tbsp, 16g	0.5	0	3	40	170
caviar, red, 1tbsp, 16g	0.5	0	3	40	170
clams, 100g	0	N	2	81	340
cockles, raw, 100g	0	0	0	48	200
cod, baked, 100g	0	0	1	76	320
cod, grilled, 100g	0	0	2	95	400
cod, poached, 100g	0	0	2	95	400
cod, smoked, simmered, 1 fillet, 195g	0	0	1.5	89	375
crab, all varieties, 90g	0	0	0.5	54	230
crab, canned in brine, 145g	2	0	1	88	370
eel, 85g	0	0	12.5	190	800
eel, smoked, 100g	10	0	13	167	700
fish ball, boiled, 1, 50g	2	0	0.5	37	155
fish paste, 1tbsp, 20g	2	0	1.5	31	130
fish roe, black, 1tbsp, 20g	0	0	1	18	75
fish roe, red, 1tbsp, 20g	0	0	1.5	30	125
fish, steamed, 1 small fillet, 85g	0	0	2.5	105	440
flake, crumbed & fried, 1 fillet, 165g	10.5	+	8.5	293	1230
flake, steamed, 1 fillet, 150g	0	0	0	187	785
flathead, fried, 1 fillet, 104g	3.5	0	7	183	770
flathead, steamed, 1 fillet, 85g	0	0	1	96	405
flounder, 100g	0	0	1	67	280
garfish, 100g	0	0	2	93	390
gernfish, 1 fillet, 175g	0	0	27	393	1650

TUNA An oily fish, tuna is a good source of vitamin D and omega-3 fatty acids. Sushi and sashimi are a delicious, low-fat way to consume very fresh fish.

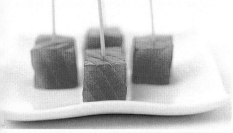

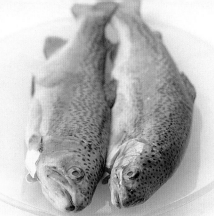

SEAFOOD – FRESH FISH

Nutritionists recommend eating at least two portions of fish, one of which should be an oily fish, each week. Fish is an excellent, low-fat source of vitamins, minerals and protein. Oily fish, such as salmon and mackerel, also contain omega-3 fatty acids, which may help to reduce the risk of arteries clotting.

TROUT An oily fish that contains omega-3 fatty acids. It is delicious baked or cooked under the grill.

RECIPE For a low-fat supper, marinate a tuna steak in ginger, lime juice, honey and a little soy sauce for 30 minutes. Chargrill, then serve with steamed rice and stir-fried vegetables.

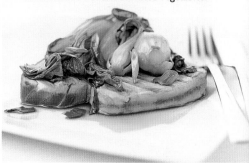

SNAPPER A white fish that is low in fat and high in vitamin B. It has a subtle flavour and is a good fish to use for steaming, baking or grilling.

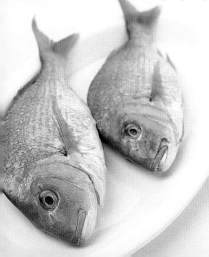

SALMON A well-known oily fish high in omega-3 fatty acids and protein. Salmon is delicious simply poached or baked and served with lemon or dill.

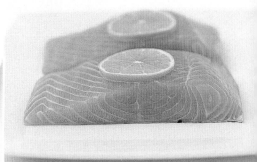

FOOD	CARB	FIBRE	FAT	ENERGY	
	g	g	g	kcal	kJ

SEAFOOD CONT.

FOOD	CARB	FIBRE	FAT	kcal	kJ
groper, 100g	0	0	1	86	360
gumard, 100g	0	0	2	86	390
haddock, smoked, 1 small fillet, 85g	0	0	1	8	35
herring, canned, drained, 125g	10	0	22.5	315	1325
jewfish (mulloway), steamed,					
1 fillet, 145g	0	0	4	128	540
kamaboko, 100g	0	0	1	52	220
kingfish, 100g	0	0	3	105	440
leatherjacket, 100g	0	0	2	93	390
lemon sole, 1 small fillet, 85g	0	0	2	79	330
ling, 100g	0	0	2	93	390
lobster, boiled, 165g	0	0	1.5	159	670
lumpfish roe, 10g	0	0	1	12	50
mackerel, 100g	0	0	16	221	930
mullet, steamed, 1 fillet, 74g	0	0	3.5	99	415
mussels, 100g	0	0	2	87	365
mullet, steamed, 1 fillet, 74g	0	0	3.5	99	415
mussels, 100g	0	0	2	87	365
mussels, smoked, canned in oil, drained, 100g	4.5	0	10.5	193	810
ocean perch, 1 fillet, 120g	0	0	2.5	112	470
octopus, 100g	0	0	1	69	290
oysters, raw, 10, 60g	0.5	0	2.5	72	305
oysters, smoked, canned in oil, drained, 10, 60g	0.5	0	7	124	520
parrot fish, 100g	0	0	2	93	390
perch, 100g	0	0	1	86	360
pike, 100g	0	0	1	88	370
pilchards, 150g	0	0	3.5	157	660
pilchards, canned in tomato sauce, 225g	2	+	29	430	1805
prawn cutlets, fried, 3, 75g	15	+	12	218	915
prawns, garlic, 100g	2.5	+	7.5	121	510
prawns, king, cooked, 100g	0	0	1	104	435
prawns, school, steamed, 150g	0	0	1.5	114	480
redfish, 100g	0	0	2	93	390
salmon, canned in brine, drained, 100g	0	0	9.5	171	720
salmon, patty mix, 100g	0	0	7.5	202	850
salmon, pink, canned in brine, drained, 100g	0	0	6.5	146	615
salmon, raw, 100g	0	0	12	181	760
salmon, red, canned in brine, drained, 100g	0	0	12	194	815
salmon, roe, 1tbsp, 10g	0	0	1	12	50
salmon, smoked, 50g	0	0	2.5	67	280
sardines, fresh, 100g	0	0	2	67	280
sardines, canned in oil, drained, 100g	0	0	15.5	226	950
sardines, canned in tomato sauce, 100g	1	Tr	13	190	800
scallops, steamed, 160g	1	0	2.5	168	705
scampi, 100g	0	0	2	107	450
scampi, crumbed, fried, 2, 100g	0	1	17.5	314	1320
sea bream, 100g	0	0	5.5	138	580

SELENIUM Shellfish contain the trace mineral selenium, a powerful antioxidant that may protect against disease, and have anti-ageing properties.

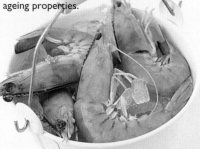

Although high in nutrients, shellfish also have a reputation for being high in cholesterol. However, cholesterol is present in all animals, and though some shellfish can have a high level, the fact that they are so low in fat, (on average less than 2%), means that they are one of the healthiest forms of protein.

RECIPE For a low-fat dinner, marinate peeled raw prawns in garlic, lime juice, macadamia oil and pepper. Grill and serve with a low-fat yoghurt and diced watermelon dressing.

OYSTERS Their reputed aphrodisiac quality can be attributed to the fact that oysters have the highest zinc content of any food, a mineral needed for growth and sexual development.

VITAMIN B Shellfish are full of Vitamin B12 which is vital for the growth of new cells and tissues and for the function of the nervous system.

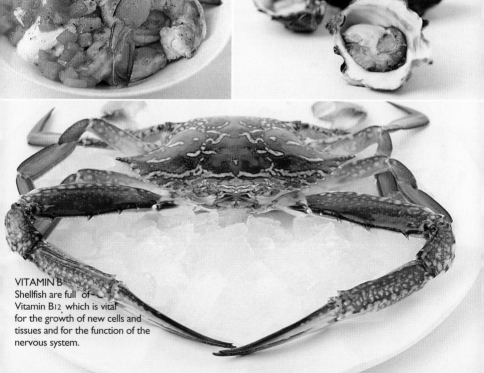

FOOD	CARB	FIBRE	FAT	ENERGY	
	g	g	g	kcal	kJ
SEAFOOD CONT.					
sea perch, 100g	0	0	1	86	360
sea trout, 100g	0	0	2	93	390
shark, 100g	0	0	1	100	420
snapper, steamed, 100g	0	0	2.5	121	510
sole, 100g	0	0	1	81	340
squid, boiled, steamed, 100g	0	0	1	79	330
squid rings, fried, 125g	8.5	0	12	257	1080
trout, coral, grilled, 100g	0	0	2	93	390
trout, rainbow, steamed, 100g	0	0	6	155	650
trout, smoked, 100g	0	0	5	136	570
tuna, canned in brine/water,					
drained, 190g	0	0	5	234	985
tuna, canned in oil, drained, 250g	0	0	28	450	1890
tuna, steamed, 100g	0	0	3	119	500
whiting, all varieties, 100g	0	0	1	93	390
SEAWEED					
raw, average all types, 10g	Tr	1.2	0	1	4
SEEDS					
poppy, 1tbsp	2	+	4	46	195
pumpkin, 50g	5	2.6	7	155	650
sesame, 1tbsp	0	0.8	7	76	320
sunflower, 1tbsp	0.5	0.9	8	88	370
SEMOLINA cooked, 1 bowl, 245g	15.5	+	0	75	315
SHALLOT 25g	N	0.3	0	6	25
SNACK FOOD (see also CORN CHIPS)					
bacon rings, 1 packet, 25g	N	0	6,5	124	520
burger rings,1 packet, 50g	0	1	13	249	1045
cheese & bacon balls, 1 packet, 50g	N	N	17	265	1115
cheese twists, 1 packet, 50g	30	0.5	13	249	1045
cheese potato puff type, 1 packet, 50g	30	0.5	15	258	1085
popcorn, microwave, 1 pack, 100g	4	1	2	32	135
potato crisps, plain, 1 large packet, 50g	25	2.6	15	249	1045
potato crisps, 1 large packet, 50g	N	2.6	16	250	1050
potato crisps, lite, 1 packet, 50g	30	3	15	258	1085
potato crisps,					
average all flavours, 50g	N	2.6	18	282	1185
potato twists, plain, 1 packet, 50g	N	1.3	17	258	1085
pork rind, crackling, 1 packet, 30g	N	0.1	8.5	145	610
prawn crackers, 5, 30g	N	0	2	45	190
pretzels-type, 10g	6.5	+	0.5	37	155
sesame seed bar, 1, 45g	20	+	12	167	700
SNAIL cooked, 2, 30g	N	0	0.5	29	120
SOFT DRINKS – CARBONATED					
(see also CORDIAL, SPORTS DRINKS AND WATER)					
cola, 375ml	39	0	0	150	630
diet cola, 375ml	1	0	0	1	5
dry ginger ale, 375ml	28	0	0	124	520

SOFT DRINKS These tend to be high in sugar and low in nutrients, and should therefore not be consumed on a regular basis. Their high sugar content also means high consumption can lead to dental caries. Small bottles of mineral water are equally easy to carry around, as are 'diet' soft drinks – although these do contain artificial sweeteners such as saccharin.

DIET SOFT DRINKS Sweetened with artificial sweeteners, such as saccharin, these drinks may be suitable for people watching their weight or suffering from diabetes. However, mineral water is a healthier option.

COLA With 8–10 teaspoons of sugar per can, these drinks are high in calories. Cola also contains significant quantities of caffeine.

FLAVOURED MINERAL WATER These usually have fruit juice added. They can have a comparable sugar content to a glass of cola or lemonade.

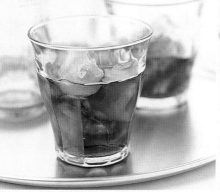

MINERAL WATER The bottles offer a portable alternative to soda water for quenching your thirst. Plain soda waters and mineral waters are free of calories.

RECIPE Combine pineapple juice, chilled camomile tea and soda water to make a delicious fruit-based soft drink.

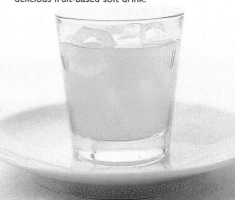

FOOD	CARB g	FIBRE g	FAT g	ENERGY kcal	kJ
SOFT DRINKS – CARBONATED CONT.					
dry ginger ale, diet, 375ml	1	0	0	4	15
orangeade, 275ml	48	0	0	194	815
orangeade, diet, 375ml	1	0	0	2	10
lemonade, 375ml	40	0	0	159	670
lemonade, diet, 375ml	1	0	0	4	15
pineapple & grapefruit flavoured, 375ml	45	0	0	161	675
diet, 375ml	1	0	0	6	25
lemon & lime flavoured, 375ml	40	0	0	179	750
lime flavoured, 375ml	40	0	0	150	630
diet, 375ml	1	0	0	4	15
tonic water, 250ml	0	0	0	82	345
SORBET lemon, 50g	7	0	0	62	260
SOUP					
chicken, low calorie, 220ml	8	N	1	50	210
condensed, beef broth, 220ml	12.5	N	2.5	81	340
condensed, creamy chicken, 220ml	12	N	6	120	505
condensed, creamy chicken & corn, 220ml	14.5	N	7	131	550
condensed, creamy chicken & mushroom, 220ml	15	N	0	70	295
condensed, creamy chicken & vegetable, natural, 215ml	10.5	N	8	139	585
condensed, creamy mushroom, 1 serving, 215ml	7	N	8	139	585
condensed, pumpkin, 1 serving, 215ml	13	N	4	96	403
condensed, creamy minestrone, 1 serving, 215ml	15	N	0.5	74	310
condensed, creamy potato & leek, 215ml	12	N	13	180	755
condensed, minestrone, 220ml	15	+	0	70	295
condensed, mushroom, 220ml	13	N	6.5	126	530
condensed, pea & ham, 220ml	15	+	0.5	94	395
condensed, tomato, 1 serving, 220ml	12	+	0.5	57	240
instant, chicken noodle, lite, 1 mug, 200ml	5	N	0.5	29	120
instant, chicken & vegetable, 1 mug, 200ml	14	N	0	60	250
instant, chunky chicken, 1 serving, 1 mug, 250ml,	31	N	3	167	700
instant, creamy cauliflower & cheese, 1 mug, lite, 200ml	9	N	1	45	190
instant, mushroom & chives, 1 mug, lite, 200ml	5.5	N	1.5	38	160
instant, pea & ham supreme, 1 mug, lite, 200ml	9.5	N	1	55	230
instant pumpkin & vegetable, 1 mug, lite, 200ml	9	N	0.5	40	170
minestrone, reduced calorie, 220ml	10	+	0	50	210
tomato, reduced calorie, 220ml	11	1.5	0	50	210
vegetable, reduced calorie, 220ml	9	1.5	0.5	48	200
SPAGHETTI (see also PASTA)					
canned, bolognaise, 130g	12.5	1.3	0.5	68	285
canned, tomato sauce, 130g	16.5	1	1.3	87	365
canned, tomato sauce & cheese, 130g	16.5	+	1	82	345
SPICES average all types, 1 tsp	0	N	0	9	40

SPICES Just like herbs, spices are used in such small quantities that they usually add little nutritional value to our diet. However, adding flavourful and fragrant spices to your food can allow you to use a lighter hand with the salt and cooking oil. Spices have also been renowned for their medicinal properties for centuries.

GINGER May help digestion, and when chewed or made into tea, can be a good relief for morning sickness.

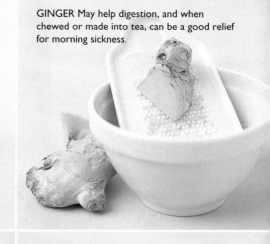

CHILLIS A spicy meal can make the eyes water and the nose run – a good way to bring relief from the blocked airways of a heavy cold.

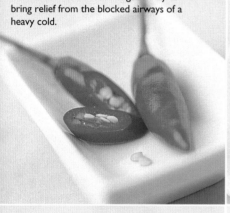

GARLIC This contains a compound called allinin, thought to help reduce blood cholesterol levels. Its pungent taste and smell make it a great flavouring to add to low-fat dishes.

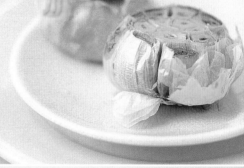

SWEET SPICE Cinnamon, star anise and cardamom are spices that can be used to add flavour to sweet dishes. Infuse in milk, or in a syrup, to poach fruit.

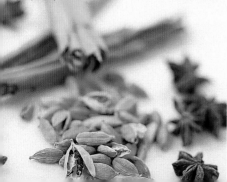

RECIPE For low-fat spicy prawns, marinate peeled and deveined raw prawns in grated ginger, crushed garlic, a finely chopped red chilli and lime juice. Thread onto skewers and barbecue or grill.

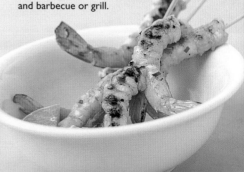

FOOD	CARB	FIBRE	FAT	ENERGY	
	g	g	g	kcal	kJ
SPINACH					
cooked, 35g	0.3	0.7	0	7	28
frozen, cooked, 35g	0.2	0.7	0	7	28
raw, 35g	0.5	0.7	0	9	37
SPORTS DRINKS					
isotonic type, 500ml	36	0	0	150	630
isotonic type, lite, 500ml	N	0	0	144	605
glucose type, 300ml	58	0	0	151	635
glucose type, lite, 500ml	N	0	0	100	420
SPREADS (see also HONEY AND JAM)					
almond spread, 100g	19	+	54	571	2400
cheddar cheese, 1tbsp	0	0	5	60	250
cheddar cheese, light, 1tbsp	1.5	0	3.5	48	200
gherkin, 1tbsp	9.5	+	0	57	240
lemon-flavoured, 1tbsp	13	0	1	59	250
marmalade, orange, 1tbsp	9	0	0	34	145
nut and chocolate, 1tbsp	N	0	6	105	440
peanut butter, crunchy, 1tbsp	3.5	1.2	10.5	125	525
peanut butter, crunchy lite, 1tbsp	6	+	7.5	112	470
peanut butter, smooth, 1tbsp	2.6	1	10.5	125	525
peanut butter, smooth lite, 1tbsp	6	+	7.5	112	470
pickles, low-calorie, 1tbsp	N	0	0	8	35
sandwich spread, 1tbsp	6	0.2	2.5	47	195
vegemite, 1tsp	0.5	0	0	8	35
yeast extract, 1tsp	Tr	0	0	8	35
SPRING ONION raw, 12g	0.5	0	0	2	10
SPROUTS					
alfalfa seeds, sprouted, raw, 100g	4	+	0.5	29	120
lentils, sprouted, raw, 100g	22	+	0.5	106	445
mung beans, sprouted, raw, 100g	4	1.5	0.5	31	131
radish seeds, sprouted, raw, 100g	3.5	+	2.5	43	180
soya beans, sprouted, raw, 100g	9.5	+	6.5	121	510
wheat seeds, sprouted, raw, 100g	42.5	+	1.5	198	830
SQUASH					
acorn, baked, 70g	9	2.2	0	39	165
butternut, baked, 70g	5	1	0	22	94
STAR FRUIT (CARAMBOLA)					
raw, 100g	7.3	1.3	0	32	136
STOCK CUBES all varieties, 1, 5g	1	0	0,5	11	45
STOCK POWDER all varieties, 1tbsp	2	0	0.5	19	80
STRAWBERRIES					
canned in syrup, 100g	17	0.7	0	65	279
raw, 100g	6	1.1	0	27	113
STUFFING average, small serving, 30g	6.5	0.5	2.5	56	235
SUET MIX 100g	10	0	90	807	3390

ISOTONIC This means that the drink contains the same concentration of carbohydrates as blood, so the carbohydrates can be easily absorbed and blood sugar levels topped up.

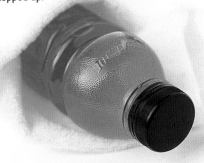

SUGAR Sports drinks do not generally contain less sugar than other soft drinks. In fact, they are often high in calories and sugars.

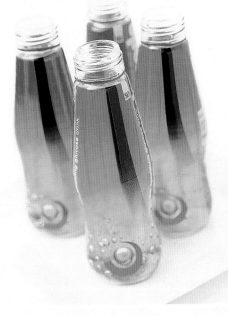

SPORTS DRINKS Many people

believe sports drinks are more 'healthy' than other soft drinks, yet they do contain a lot of sugars such as dextrose and glucose syrup, which are high in calories. Many of the drinks provide mineral salts, which are lost through sweating, but only highly trained athletes are likely to need this additional source.

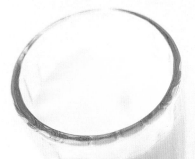

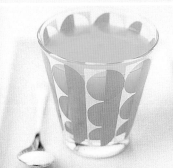

RECIPE People who engage in a lot of exercise could mix orange juice with water and a tiny amount of salt and sugar as a healthy alternative.

SODIUM Sports drinks have added sodium to speed up fluid absorption. Salt lost through perspiration can be replaced through food or even a glass of milk.

FOOD	CARB g	FIBRE g	FAT g	ENERGY kcal	kJ
SUGAR					
average, 1 tsp	5	0	0	19	80
any type, 1 tbsp	17	0	0	64	270
icing, 1 tbsp	20	0	0	76	320
SULTANAS dried, 1 tbsp	13.5	0.5	0	55	230
SUSHI					
Californian roll, 5 pieces	N	N	2	139	585
inari (bean curd pouch with rice), 85g	N	N	2	130	545
nigiri, 30g	N	N	0.5	30	125
SWEDE					
peeled, boiled, 150g	3	1	0	16	69
SWEET POTATO					
peeled, boiled, 100g	20.5	2.3	0	84	358
raw, 1, 235g	50	5.6	0	56	237
SWEETS (see also CHOCOLATE)					
boiled, 1	5	0	0	15	65
butterscotch, 1	5.5	0	0	24	100
caramels, 1	4	0	0	24	100
fruit gums, 30g	27	0	0	8	35
fudge, 2 pieces, 35g	28.5	0	4.5	155	650
jaffas, 55g	N	0	18	245	1030
jelly babies, 1	3.5	0	0	15	65
jellybeans, 1	3	0	0	11	45
liquorice allsorts, 100g	77	2	5.2	349	1483
liquorice pieces, 100g	65	1.9	1.4	278	1185
peppermints, 1 packet	N	0	0	84	355
marshmallows, 1 packet, 85g	68	0	0	283	1190
sesame seed bar, 45g	N	+	12	167	700
sherbet lemons, 1	N	0	0	20	85
toffees, 1	3.5	0	0.5	20	85
SWISS CHARD raw, 30g	1	N	0	6	25
TACO					
with meat & bean sauce, 1 serving, 180g	N	+	14	231	970
TAHINI paste, 1 tbsp	0.2	1.6	11.8	121	510
TAMARILLO (TREE TOMATO)					
raw, peeled, 90g	4	+	0	24	100
TANGERINE raw, peeled, 100g	8	1.3	0	35	147
TAPIOCA cooked, 1 bowl, 265g	18.5	0.3	0	75	315
TEA					
for each teaspoon of sugar in tea, add ...	5	0	0	19	80
black, no sugar, 1 cup, 250 ml	Tr	0	0	Tr	Tr
with whole milk, 1 cup, 250ml	1	0	1	18	75
with skim milk, 1 cup, 250ml	1.5	0	0	13	55
TINNED FRUITS (see also FRUIT SALAD)					
peach & mango in syrup, 133g	12	1	0	56	235
sliced peaches in syrup, 133g	18	1.2	0	71	300
fruit salad in syrup, 125g	15	1.5	0	59	250

SUGAR

Most healthy eating advice today focuses on eating less fat and saturated fat. However, consuming too many sugary foods and drinks can lead to both tooth decay and weight gain. Sugar is sometimes associated with 'empty calories' as it provides only energy and has no nutritional benefit.

HIDDEN SUGAR Most of the sugar in our diet comes from the sugar in confectionery, cakes, biscuits, soft drinks and other processed foods.

HONEY This contains as many calories as sugar and is just as likely to cause tooth decay.

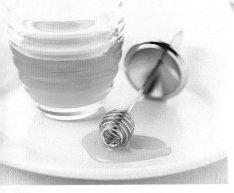

SOFT BROWN SUGAR This is in fact white sugar that has been coloured and flavoured with sugar cane molasses. It has no nutritional benefits over white sugar.

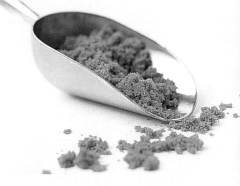

ARTIFICIAL SWEETENERS These provide no calories and offer a sugar substitute for those trying to reduce their sugar intake.

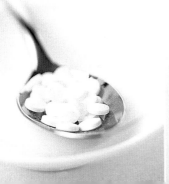

MAPLE SYRUP Like honey, syrup contains as many calories as sugar and can cause tooth decay when eaten to excess.

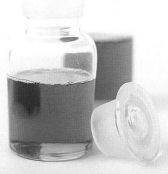

FOOD	CARB	FIBRE	FAT	ENERGY	
	g	g	g	kcal	kJ
TOFU					
dessert, fruit-flavoured, 100g	12.5	N	1	67	280
firm, 100g	0.7	N	4.2	73	304
fried, 100g	2	N	17.7	261	1086
silken, 100g	3	0	2.5	55	230
tofu burgers, 100g	N	N	9.5	174	730
tofu veggie burgers, 100g	N	N	9.5	174	730
soya burger mix, 30g	26	+	1.3	168	704
TOMATO					
canned in juice, 250g	7.5	1.7	0.2	40	172
juice, 250g	7.5	1.5	0	35	155
purée, 1tbsp	2	0.6	0	13	55
cherry, 100g	3	1	0.4	18	76
raw, 1 large, 100g	3.1	1	0	17	73
sundried, natural, 5 pieces, 10g	5.5	+	0.5	26	110
sundried, in oil, drained, 3 pieces, 10g	2.5	+	1.5	21	90
TOPPING					
caramel, 1tbsp	11	0	0	45	190
chocolate, 1tbsp	12.5	0	0	54	225
strawberry, 1tbsp	9	0	0	39	165
TORTILLA					
corn, 1, 50g	24.5	N	4.5	152	640
wheat flour, 1, 50g	30	1.2	0.5	131	557
TRIFLE commercial, made with cream,					
1 serving, 120g	23	0.6	11	199	837
TURKEY					
baked, lean. 120g	0	0	5	186	780
breast, no skin, 80g	0	0	3.5	20	83
breast, with skin, basted, 100g	0	0	8	145	610
1 slice	0	0	4	149	625
cooked meat, 100g	0	0	11.5	167	700
roast, dark meat, 100g	0	0	4	133	560
roast, light meat, 100g	0	0	1.5	133	560
roast, with skin, 100g	0	0	6.5	170	715
salami, 100g	0	0	4	149	625
smoked, 75g	0	0	1	80	335
TURNIP peeled, boiled, 240g	4.8	4.5	0	29	121
VEAL					
boneless, unspecified cut, lean, 1, 190g	0	0	5	282	1185
boneless, unspecified cut, untrimmed, 1, 200g	0	0	8	319	1340
cutlet crumbed & fried, 1	0	0	5	174	730
forequarter steak lean, 119g	0	0	6	329	1380
forequarter steak, untrimmed, 1, 200g	0	0	10.5	373	1565
heart, baked, 100g	0	0	6	181	760
kidney, grilled, 100g	0	0	5.51	167	700
leg, lean, baked, 2 slices, 44g	0	0	0.5	54	225
leg, untrimmed, baked, 2 slices, 45g	0	0	0.5	64	270
leg, steak, lean, fried, 1, 85g	0	0	2.5	131	550

TOFU Made from soya beans, these are low in fat, high in calcium and excellent sources of protein for vegetarians. All soya products contain phytoestrogens, which are hormone-like substances in plants. Although opinion is divided, some studies suggest that these substances may help to protect women from breast cancer and symptoms of the menopause.

FIRM TOFU This holds its shape well when cooked. It can be marinated and then fried or grilled, or cut into pieces and added to curries. Store in water in the refrigerator.

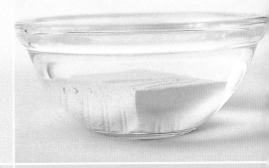

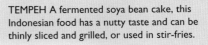

SILKEN TOFU This soft tofu can be blended and used instead of dairy products in dips, ice creams or cheesecakes. It is also wonderful as a simple dessert sweetened with bananas and maple syrup.

TEMPEH A fermented soya bean cake, this Indonesian food has a nutty taste and can be thinly sliced and grilled, or used in stir-fries.

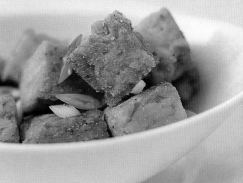

RECIPE Marinate thick slices of firm tofu in a mixture of grated ginger and soy sauce for several hours. Fry, grill or add to a stir-fry.

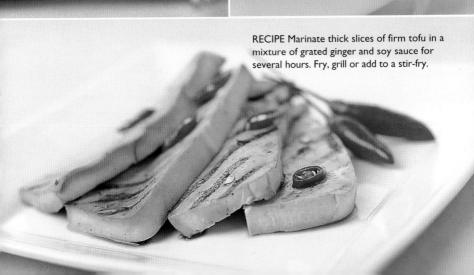

FOOD	CARB	FIBRE	FAT	ENERGY	
	g	g	g	kcal	kJ

VEAL CONT.

FOOD	CARB	FIBRE	FAT	ENERGY	
leg steak, untrimmed, fried, 1, 100g	0	0	4	159	670
liver, grilled, 85g	1.5	0	7	159	670
loin chop, lean, baked or grilled, 1, 50g	0	0	1.5	73	305
loin chop, untrimmed, baked or grilled, 1, 55g	0	0	2.5	88	370
schnitzel, fried, 1, 85g	8.5	N	23	287	1205
shank, lean, simmered, 1, 80g	0	0	2	117	490
shank, untrimmed, simmered, 1, 90g	0	0	6	160	670
shoulder steak, lean, grilled, 1 small, 50g	0	0	1.5	73	305
shoulder steak, untrimmed, grilled, 1 small, 55g	0	0	2.5	84	355
VEGETABLE JUICE, average, 250ml	11	0	0.5	51	215

VEGETABLE JUICE, average, 250ml

VEGETABLES (see INDIVIDUAL VEGETABLES)

FOOD	CARB	FIBRE	FAT	ENERGY	
VENISON roast, 100g	0	0	5.5	157	660

VINEGAR

FOOD	CARB	FIBRE	FAT	ENERGY	
apple cider, 100ml	6	0	0	14	60
unspecified, 100ml	15.5	0	0	21	90
white, 1tbsp	0	0	0	4	15

WAFFLES

FOOD	CARB	FIBRE	FAT	ENERGY	
frozen, 1 square, 35g	13.5	1	2.5	88	370
homemade, 1 round, 75g	24.5	2	10.5	218	915

WATER (see also SOFT DRNKS)

FOOD	CARB	FIBRE	FAT	ENERGY	
plain mineral, soda, tap, 1 glass, 250g	0	0	0	0	0
bottled, average, all varieties, 1 glass, 250g	0	0	0	0	0

WATER CHESTNUTS

FOOD	CARB	FIBRE	FAT	ENERGY	
canned, drained, 40g	3.5	+	0.5	19	80
raw, 5, 50g	12	+	0	49	205
WATERCRESS raw, 32g	0.5	0.5	0	6	25
WHEATGERM 1tbsp	1.5	0.8	0.5	17	70
YAM baked or boiled 100g	37.5	1.7	0.4	153	651

YEAST

FOOD	CARB	FIBRE	FAT	ENERGY	
dried, bakers, compressed, 1 sachet, 7g	0.5	N	0	8	35
dried, brewers, 1 sachet, 7g	0.5	N	0.5	19	80

YOGHURT

FOOD	CARB	FIBRE	FAT	ENERGY	
acidophilus, live, low-fat, 100ml	11	0	0	56	235
acidophilus, plain, 100ml	8	0	3.3	24	100
bio type, acidophilus, low-fat, honey & strawberry, 100ml	13	0	3	100	420
black cherry, with live cultures, 100ml	17	0	4	104	435
drinking, apricot, 250ml	31	N	5	190	800
drinking, 100ml	13	0	1	81	340
drinking, swiss type, vanilla, 250ml	31.5	N	5	184	775
drinking, vitamin-enriched, 250ml	24	N	5	139	585
drinking, fruit, 250ml	31.8	N	5	190	800
frozen, fruit, 100ml	20	0	5	132	555
frozen, fruit yoghurt stick, raspberry, strawberry, 85ml	20	0	5	132	555
frozen, low-fat, 100ml	N	0	3	114	480
frozen, low-fat, flavoured, 100ml	22	0	0	83	350

VEGETABLES Try to eat at least five portions of vegetables and fruit each day. Vegetables are high in fibre and are packed with vitamins and minerals. Choose from fresh, frozen, raw and canned varieties, but bear in mind that vegetables lose vitamin C if stored for a long time or are cooked for too long in a lot of water.

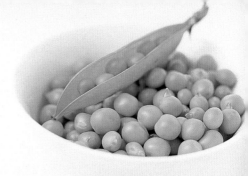

PEAS Fresh peas are delicious, but are not always available. Frozen peas are convenient and a good source of vitamins and fibre.

BROCCOLI A rich source of vitamin C and folic acid, broccoli is also associated with antioxidant properties.

CORN An excellent source of vitamin C, a good source of fibre and a moderate source of thiamin and niacin.

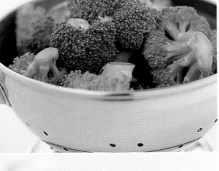

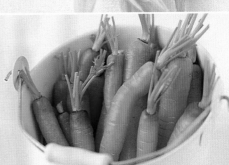

RECIPE To prepare vegetables without adding fat, steam some vegetables, drizzle with lemon juice and sprinkle with black pepper.

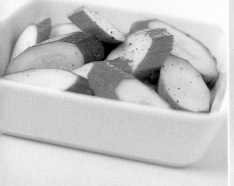

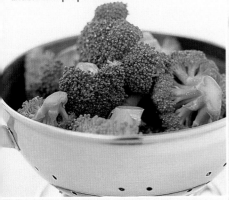

CARROTS Rich in beta carotene, an antioxidant that may help prevent chronic diseases such as heart disease. Carrots are the best source as there is no evidence that beta carotene supplements have any benefit.

FOOD	CARB	FIBRE	FAT	ENERGY	
	g	g	g	kcal	kJ
YOGHURT CONT.					
frozen, low-fat, low sugar, 1 cone	N	0	0	45	190
frozen, fat-free, honey, 1 cone	N	0	0	109	460
frozen, reduced-fat honey, 1 cone	N	0	0	90	380
frozen, strawberry, 85ml	N	0	4	127	535
fruit cocktail, diet lite, 100ml	13	0	0.2	92	385
honey, dairy style, 100ml	11.5	0	7	132	555
kiwifruit & mango, diet lite, 100ml	13.6	0	0.2	94	395
lemon, cultured, 100ml	15	0	0	82	345
low-fat, berry, diet lite, 100ml	15	0	1	87	365
low-fat, berry fruits, live, diet lite, 100ml	7	0	0	43	180
low-fat, fruit salad, blueberry, cherry, diet lite, bio type, 100ml	7	0	0	43	180
low-fat, passionfruit, 100ml	16	0	0	89	375
low-fat peach, diet lite, bio type, 100ml	6.5	0	0	42	175
low-fat, peach & mango, diet lite, 100ml	15	0	2	194	815
low-fat, plain. dairy type, 100ml	6	0	0	51	215
low-fat, strawberry, diet lite, bio type, 100ml	6.5	0	0	42	175
low-fat, summer fruits, diet lite, 100ml	16	0	1	93	390
low-fat, vanilla, diet lite, bio type, 100ml	6	0	0	40	170
low-fat, vanilla, fruit & nut, diet lite, 100ml	16	0	1	40	170
plain, bio type, 100ml	5	0	4.5	95	400
plain, dairy type, 100ml	6	0	8	120	505
plain, skim milk natural, 100ml	7	0	0.1	51	215
plain, swiss style, creamy custard, 100ml	1	0	4.5	107	450
plain, traditional, dairy type, 100ml	6.5	0	35	77	325
soft serve, 100ml	16.5	0	0	80	335
soft serve, low-fat, average	N	0	0	80	335
soft serve, natural, 100ml	24	0	2	142	595
soft serve, fat-free, 100ml	4.5	0	0	21	90
strawberry delight, 125ml	20	0	4	136	570
vanilla, cultured, 100ml	19	0	4	114	480
yoghurt, cultured, 65ml	11	0	0	46	195
yoghurt, baby type, banana/vanilla, 100ml	N	0	4	107	450
yogurt, average, all flavours, 150ml	N	0	5	167	700
YORKSHIRE PUDDING					
small serve, 50g	12.3	0.5	5	104	437
ZUCCHINI					
green, boiled, 90g	1.5	1	0.5	13	55
yellow, boiled, 90g	1	1	0.5	17	70

YOGHURT

The fat content of yoghurt will largely depend on whether it is made from whole or skimmed milk. It is always an excellent source of calcium and B-group vitamins. Although low-fat varieties make a healthy dessert, they may still be quite high in calories, as they often contain added sugars.

NATURAL YOGHURT The name says it all, it has no added flavours or colouring and is simply milk with a starter culture added. Select a low-fat variety.

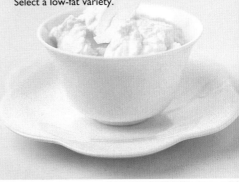

FRUIT YOGHURT Must contain at least 5% fruit. Manufacturers may also add flavours, colours, sugar and thickeners. A fruit-flavoured yoghurt often contains fruit flavourings, rather than actual fruit.

DIET YOGHURT These are usually made with low-fat yoghurt sweetened artificially so that they are also low in sugar. These tend to be the lowest in calories of all the yoghurts.

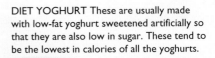

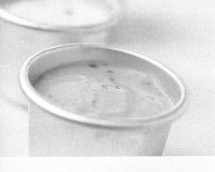

RECIPE Make your own flavoured yoghurt by adding honey, vanilla essence, puréed fruit or berries to low-fat natural yoghurt.

ACIDOPHILUS A live culture that can be added to yoghurt. There is evidence that it may help to restore levels of healthy bacteria in the gut after an infection or antibiotics.

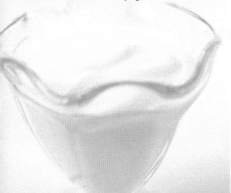

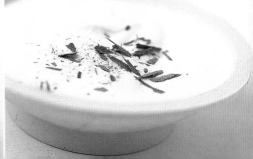

VITAMIN AND MINERAL
Counter

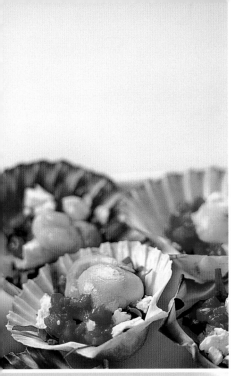

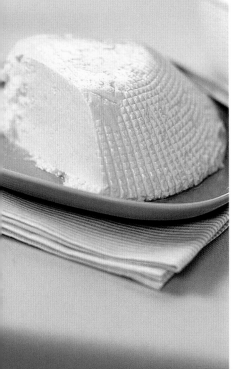

HOW TO USE THE TABLES

This section contains charts and tables, one for each vitamin and most minerals, listing foods that are good sources of these nutrients. Each chart states the adult RNI (where applicable) and lists the average amount of vitamin or mineral contained in 100g of the edible part of the food. Vitamins and minerals are only present in foods (and needed in the body) in small amounts, for example, milligrams (mg) or micrograms (mcg).

The tables will help you estimate the nutrient content of your diet and thus improve your eating habits by making better food choices and meeting the RNI. All nutrient values are for the raw, uncooked food unless otherwise stated. Foods at the top of the lists contain relatively high amounts of the nutrient per 100g. Although not all of these foods are eaten in large amounts, such as yeast extract or wheat bran, they can make a valuable contribution to your nutrient intake if eaten regularly. On the other hand, some of the foods at the bottom of the lists (which contain lower levels of the particular nutrient) may be eaten in larger amounts, such as potatoes and pasta, and therefore also make a significant contribution to your nutrient intake. Potatoes, for example, account for about 35 per cent of the vitamin C intake in the UK. Some of the recipe ideas and suggestions accompanying the lists will give you examples of how to incorporate these foods into your daily diet.

VITAMINS AND MINERALS are naturally occurring substances that are essential to life. They are only needed in small amounts, but have powerful effects essential to health and well-being. They are obtained by eating a wide variety of different foods combined to make a healthy, balanced diet.

VITAMINS

These are micronutrients required for the normal functioning of all our organs, as well as functions such as growth, reproduction and tissue repair. Although they do not provide energy, they are needed for the release of energy from the macronutrients, carbohydrates, fats and proteins. With the exception of vitamins D and K, vitamins can't be made by the body and so have to be obtained through the food we eat. Vitamins can be broadly divided into two groups: fat-soluble and water-soluble.

FAT-SOLUBLE VITAMINS: These include vitamins A, D, E and K. Each have unique functions (see page 112) and occur generally in foods with a substantial fat content, such as oils, dairy products, meat, fish, nuts and grains. Because fat-soluble vitamins can be stored in the body for long periods of time, consuming large quantities can be toxic. They are fairly stable during cooking and processing, but can be destroyed by exposure to air, light or high temperatures.

WATER-SOLUBLE VITAMINS: These include vitamin C and eight B-group vitamins. These dissolve in water and so excessive amounts are generally removed from the body in the urine, although large quantities of some B vitamins (B6 and B12) can still cause toxicity problems. These vitamins can be lost in the washing, soaking or boiling of foods and may be destroyed by light or high temperatures.

MINERALS

These are essential to many processes, including maintaining the body's fluid balance and the structure of hormones, bones and teeth, the regulation of blood pressure, wound healing and the activity of muscles and nerves. Minerals cannot be made by the body, so we have to obtain them from our diet. They can be divided into two groups: major minerals and trace minerals.

MAJOR MINERALS: These include calcium, sodium, potassium, magnesium, phosphorus, chlorine and sulphur. They are classed as 'major' minerals because they are present in the body in greater amounts than the second category, trace elements.

TRACE ELEMENTS: These include iron, copper, zinc, manganese, selenium, iodine, chromium, fluoride and molybdenum. They each have different functions and cause individual deficiency symptoms if not eaten in sufficient quantities. Many other trace elements, such as boron, nickel and silicon are also found in the body, but the amounts we need to eat for optimum health are not really known.

Minerals tend to be more stable than vitamins, although the levels found in foods can be affected by food processing and preparation methods. The availability of minerals from the food we eat can be strongly affected by other nutrients (see table, top right). For example, dietary fibre can reduce the absorption of some minerals from food, whereas the lactose in milk can increase calcium absorption.

The absorption and functions of many minerals are interrelated, so a deficiency or excess of one can affect the absorption and function of others. This is why high doses of any mineral supplement should only be taken under strict medical supervision (see also 'Supplements', page 110).

MINERAL MATTERS

Mineral	Availability/use **enhanced** by:	Availability/use **decreased** by:
Calcium	Vitamin D Regular exercise Lactose	Very high fibre intake Oxalate from spinach and rhubarb Excessive saturated fat intake
Iron	Vitamin C	Very high fibre intake Tannin (eg. in tea) Excessive zinc
Zinc	Protein Adequate energy (calories)	Very high fibre intake Excessive alcohol Excessive iron Excessive calcium
Selenium	Vitamins A, C and E	Not applicable

HOW MUCH OF EACH MINERAL AND VITAMIN DO WE NEED?

This depends on our age, gender, body size, physical activity levels, physiological status (i.e. pregnancy, breast-feeding, illness), use of medication and lifestyle factors (such as stress, smoking, exposure to pollution, alcohol and fat intake). Scientists are also trying to find out whether people with a family history of cancer, osteoporosis, heart disease and other diseases may be able to reduce their risk of developing these diseases by consuming greater amounts of certain vitamins and minerals. However, healthy people should be able to get all the vitamins and minerals they need from a balanced and varied diet.

Dietary reference values

In 1991, the UK Department of Health published Dietary Reference Values (DRVs) for Food Energy and Nutrients for the UK. DRVs is a general term for current daily dietary recommendations. Prior to the publication of this document, Recommended Daily Amounts (or RDAs) were used. RDA values were set high compared to average requirements to ensure they covered the requirements of whole groups within the population.

Although not intended for individuals, they were often wrongly used in this way. By giving a range of intakes for energy and nutrients based on the distribution of requirements, rather than just one figure, DRVs recognise the broad range of requirements of individuals within a population.

DRV is a general term that covers:
Estimated Average Requirements (EAR). This is the average requirement of a group for a particular nutrient or energy. Many people need more, and many less than the EAR.

Reference Nutrient Intake (RNI). This is the amount of a nutrient that is sufficient for almost all individuals. This level of intake is higher than most people need.

Lower Reference Nutrient Intake (LRNI). This is the amount of a nutrient that is sufficient for only a few individuals with low needs. Most people need more than the LRNI.

Safe Intake. This is a range of intakes sufficient for almost all individuals' needs, but not high enough to cause undesirable effects. This is given for nutrients where there is currently insufficient information to estimate requirements precisely.

DRVs give a general guide to whether or not an individual's diet is likely to be nutritionally adequate. This book gives RNIs for most vitamins and minerals, as this is the level likely to be adequate for most people.

OPTIMUM INTAKES

Nutrient intake in relation to health is sometimes described in the following way: deficient, adequate, optimal, excessive, toxic. RNIs are usually set at a level to prevent deficiency. An 'optimal' intake refers to a level of intake that not only prevents deficiency, but also that may positively improve health or protect us from disease. Scientists are currently unable to calculate RNIs for optimal health and do not recommend the regular consumption of high dose vitamin and mineral supplements.

GETTING THE MOST FROM YOUR FOOD

Although we tend to think that modern foods are depleted in vitamins and minerals, supermarkets are actually full of nutritious foods – fresh, frozen and dried. Vitamins and minerals are even added to some processed foods to replace those that are lost during the manufacturing process (eg. fortified breakfast cereals and bread), or to increase the nutrient content of food (eg. some milks and fat spreads). There are ways to retain more of the nutrients in the meals you prepare:

- When you buy fresh fruit and vegetables, ensure they are as fresh as possible and eat them within a few days. Store in a cool, dark, dry place for the shortest possible time.
- To retain more vitamins, blanch and freeze fruit and vegetables from fresh.
- When preparing fruit and vegetables, cut them with a sharp knife and do not slice too finely. Where possible, try to leave the skin on. In potatoes, for example, most of the vitamin C is found just beneath the skin.

- Eat vegetables raw, or if you are going to cook them, prepare them just before cooking. Microwaving or stir-frying retains more nutrients than boiling. Cook all vegetables for the shortest time and in a small amount of water. If boiling, bring the water to the boil first, cut up the vegetables, then add them to the water. Vitamin C and B are easily destroyed during boiling. They leach out into the cooking water.
- Eat food straight away once cooked. Keeping food warm for 15 minutes, for example, could reduce the vitamin C content by 25 per cent.
- Fresh fruit and vegetables aren't always better than canned or frozen. Canned beans, for example, contain similar levels of nutrients to home-cooked dried beans; quickly reheated frozen peas contain more nutrients than overcooked (or old) fresh ones.
- Do not use bicarbonate of soda when cooking (sometimes done to help retain green colour of vegetables). It destroys vitamin C.

SUPPLEMENTS

At the moment, it's safe to say that the perfect supplement does not exist, but it is clear that a balanced diet offers many health benefits. Whole foods are a complex package of nutrients and other beneficial factors that are not found in supplements. For example, an orange contains vitamin C with carotene, folate, calcium, fibre and possibly other bio-active compounds that may protect our health. You won't get all of these elements in a vitamin C supplement. Apart from tasting better, here are some other reasons why we should get our nutrients from food rather than supplements:

- Other components in food (not present in supplements) can increase nutrient absorption in the body.
- The chemical form of a nutrient may be different from the natural form and may not be absorbed as well.

- High-dose supplements can reduce absorption of other nutrients.
- Taking excessive amounts of some nutrients may have toxic effects, or in the case of some water-soluble vitamins, the excess may just be excreted in the urine.
- Foods also contain other bio-active compounds (or phytochemicals) that have antioxidant properties and may help protect us against cancer, heart disease and diabetes.

WHEN ARE SUPPLEMENTS NEEDED?

In some circumstances, vitamin and mineral supplements may be needed to improve your health or to prevent a health problem from developing. There are two reasons why you may not get all the nutrients you need from your diet: either you don't eat enough or you don't absorb enough. Some people don't get all the nutrients they need from their diet, because they don't eat a healthy balance of foods or because they have a greater nutrient requirement (eg. during pregnancy, illness or high activity levels). Also, high intakes of fat, alcohol and certain medications can increase the body's use of certain vitamins and minerals, while some illnesses and medications prevent them from being absorbed.

While most people can get all the vitamins and minerals they need from a healthy diet, some groups of people may benefit from certain supplements:

- Folic acid is recommended for women planning to have a baby. They should take 400 mcg folic acid every day until the end of the twelfth week of pregnancy to reduce the risk of the baby being born with neural tube defects.
- Vitamin D may be needed for children under the age of four, pregnant and breast-feeding women, and people over 65 years if they don't include much meat and fish in their diet. It may also be required by people who rarely go outdoors (eg. are housebound or in residential care) or those who wear very concealing clothing.

Some young African-Caribbean children who have a very strict vegan diet, and babies, children and women from some Asian communities may need extra vitamin D.

- Vitamin drops containing vitamins A, C and D are recommended for children under the age of five as a safeguard for when their diets may be insufficient. You should start giving your baby vitamin drops (available at low cost from health centres) at six months old, if you are still breast-feeding or when your baby has less than one pint of infant formula every day. Ask your health visitor for advice.

Also, if you fit into any of the following categories, you may benefit from taking some supplements and should seek medical advice:

- Women with regular heavy periods may need iron supplements.
- If you are a heavy smoker or drinker, you may benefit from supplements eg. vitamin C and some B vitamins.
- If you are removing whole food groups from your diet due to allergy or intolerance. For example, avoiding all dairy products may mean you need extra calcium and vitamin D.
- If you have a strict vegan diet, you may need extra iron, vitamin B12 and vitamin D.
- If you have a low-calorie weight-loss diet, you may need extra iron, calcium and zinc.
- If you are taking certain long-term medications, they may interfere with the absorption of some nutrients.

If you are healthy and you want to take a supplement, choose a multi-vitamin/mineral variety, providing RNI amounts or less.

VITAMINS
FAT-SOLUBLE

	RNI	FUNCTION
VITAMIN A	Females 11+ years: 600 mcg RE*/day. Pregnancy: 700 mcg RE/day. Lactation: 950 mcg RE/day. Males 15+ years: 700 mcg RE/day. Do not exceed: 7500 mcg RE/day (females); pregnant women, see page 127; 9000 mcg RE/day (males).	For reproduction and development. Required for healthy skin, eyes and hair. Helps the body resist infection and maintains healthy mucous membranes.
VITAMIN D	No RNI except females and males 65+ years: 10 mcg/day. Pregnancy and lactation: 10 mcg/day. Vitamin D is made when skin is exposed to sunlight.	Needed for calcium and phosphorus absorption and for healthy bones and teeth.
VITAMIN E	Safe intake:+ Men above 4 mg/day. Women above 3mg/day.	Natural antioxidant, helps healing, prevents scarring. Keeps nerves and red blood cells healthy. Protects cell membranes.
VITAMIN K	Safe intake: Adults 1 mcg/kg body weight/day. Most of the body's vitamin K is synthesised by intestinal bacteria, only about 20 per cent is obtained from foods.	Called the band-aid vitamin, promotes blood clotting to stop bleeding.
OTHER FAT-SOLUBLE NUTRIENTS **ESSENTIAL FATTY ACIDS**	.Approximately 1 per cent of total energy (kj/cal) intake. No RNI	Needed for normal development and growth, and healthy skin and eyes.

* RE Dietary vitamin A (or retinol) is measured in retinol equivalents (RE) because, as well as the ready-formed vitamin A in foods of animal origin, beta carotene (sometimes called pro-vitamin A) in plant foods is converted to retinol in the body. 6 mcg of beta carotene is equivalent to 1 mcg retinol. So RE represents the retinol present in the foods plus the vitamin A that will be made in the body from the beta carotene.

DEFICIENCY SIGNS	FOOD SOURCES	SYNERGISTS	ABSORPTION INHIBITORS
Poor vision, dry scaly skin, impaired reproduction and growth, increased susceptibility to infection.	Liver, fish, eggs, dairy products (eg. milk and cheese). Yellow, orange, red and dark green vegetables contain large amounts of beta carotene eg. dried apricots, sweet potato, mangoes, carrots, spinach, watercress.	Zinc, vitamin D.	Colestipol, Cholestyramine, Epsom salts, some antibiotics, alcohol, a very low fat intake.
Muscle and bone weakness. Rickets in children. Osteomalacia in adults.	Kippers, mackerel, salmon, canned sardines, herrings, tuna, prawns, milk, butter, fortified margarines, egg yolk, fish oils.	Vitamin A, calcium and phosphorus.	Alcohol, some antibiotics, olestra, mineral oil, laxatives, some anticonvulsants.
Rare. Can occur in premature babies and people on very low-fat diets. Red blood cells may rupture, poor wound healing.	Wheat germ oil, sunflower seeds, sunflower oil, safflower oil, peanut oil, olive oil, almonds, peanuts, hazelnuts, eggs, green leafy vegetables and wholegrains.	Vitamin C.	Metals, heat, oxygen, freezing, processing, large intakes of vitamin K, Epsom salts, laxatives, senokot.
Abnormal blood clotting, haemorrhaging. Deficiency is rare in adults but can occur in newborn babies.	Green leafy vegetables (eg. broccoli, kale, Brussels sprouts, cabbage and Swiss chard), milk, liver, wheat bran, oats, vegetable oils.	Vitamin C.	Unstable to heat, freezing, warfarin, x-rays, radiation, air pollution, some antibiotics, mineral oil, laxatives, large doses of vitamin E.
Impaired vision and hearing, growth failure in infants, dry scaly skin, poor wound healing.	Oily fish, cold-pressed vegetable oils, nuts, hazelnuts, prawns, salmon, soya beans.	Vitamin E.	Not applicable.

✛ alpha-tocopherol is the most prevalent form of vitamin E, but you may see it listed as 'mixed tocopherols' on food labels and supplements.

VITAMINS
WATER-SOLUBLE

	RNI	FUNCTION
VITAMIN B1 THIAMIN	Females 15+ years: 0.8 mg/day. Pregnancy: 0.9 mg/day. Lactation: 1.0 mg/day. Males 19–50 years 1.0 mg/day. Males 51+ years 0.9 mg/day. Consuming over 3 g/day over a long period may have undesirable effects.	Needed for converting food into energy, growth in childhood and fertility in adults. Maintains healthy heart and nervous system.
VITAMIN B2 RIBOFLAVIN	Females 11+ years: 1.1 mg/day. Pregnancy: 1.4 mg/day. Lactation: 1.6 mg/day. Males 15+ years: 1.3 mg/day.	Helps the body release energy from food. Promotes growth, also needed for healthy eyes, hair, skin and nails.
VITAMIN B3 NIACIN★	Females 19–50 years: 13 mg NE/day. Females 51+ years: 12 mg NE/day. No extra needed during pregnancy. Lactation: 15 mg NE/day. Males 19–50 years: 17 mg NE/day. Males 51+ years: 16 mg/day.	Needed to release energy from food. Involved in controlling blood sugar, keeping skin healthy and maintaining healthy nervous and digestive systems.
VITAMIN B5 PANTOTHENIC ACID	No RNI. Intakes of 3–7 mg/day are considered adequate.	Helps the body release energy from food. Aids the formation of antibodies and maintains a healthy nervous system and skin.
VITAMIN B6 PYRIDOXINE	Females 15+ years: 1.2 mg/day. No extra needed during pregnancy or lactation. Males 19+ years: 1.4 mg/day. Very high intakes (between 50 mg/day and 7 g/day) have been associated with impaired function of the sensory nerves.	Essential for protein metabolism, forming red blood cells, antibodies and neurotransmitters (brain chemicals).

★ The related compounds – nicotinic acid and nicotinamide – are both called niacin. In addition to the preformed vitamin occurring in food, one of the essential amino acids tryptophan can be converted in the body to niacin. Total vitamin activity (expressed as niacin equivalent – NE) is derived from preformed vitamin plus the amount made in the body from tryptophan.

DEFICIENCY SIGNS	FOOD SOURCES	SYNERGISTS	ABSORPTION INHIBITORS
Muscle fatigue, poor concentration, irritability, depression, heart problems. Severe deficiency: beri-beri.	Yeast extract, brown rice, porridge, wheat germ, pulses, nuts, seeds, lean meats (especially pork), offal, wholegrain products, fortified breakfast cereals.	Other B vitamins, sulphur.	Can be destroyed by cooking, storage or processing. Sensitive to oxygen, heat, low-acid conditions. Alcohol, sulphur drugs, some antibiotics, antacids, tea, coffee, blueberries, red cabbage, water.
Poor wound healing, sore, watery bloodshot eyes, cracked lips and corners of the mouth, flaking skin, rash between nose and lips, confusion.	Yeast extract, milk, cheese, yoghurt, eggs, meat, offal (eg. liver), green leafy vegetables, fortified breakfast cereals.	Other B vitamins.	Destroyed by heat and light. Oral contraceptive pill, alcohol, sulphur drugs, some tranquillisers and antidepressants.
Rare. Dermatitis, nausea, diarrhoea, muscular weakness, depression, dementia. Severe deficiency: pellagra – bright red tongue, headaches.	Yeast extract, pork, chicken, beef, fish, nuts, cheese, milk, eggs, bread, potatoes, pasta, rice and fortified breakfast cereals.	Other B vitamins, especially B6, vitamin C.	B2 is the most stable B vitamin. Sulphur drugs, alcohol, food processing.
Rare and hard to diagnose. May occur in conjunction with other B deficiencies.	Dried yeast, liver, yeast extract, kidney, nuts, wheat germ, soya flour, brown rice, eggs, pulses, wholemeal bread,	Other B vitamins.	Exposure to heat. Food processing, canning, caffeine, sulphur drugs, antibiotics, alcohol.
Depression, headaches, confusion, numbness and tingling in hands and feet, anaemia, skin lesions, poor growth, decreased antibody formation (immunity).	Dried yeast, yeast extract, wholemeal bread, wheat germ, wheatbran, fortified breakfast cereals, liver, avocados, bananas, fish, meat, nuts.	Vitamins B1, B2, B5.	Exposure to heat and light. Prolonged storage, food processing, roasting and stewing meats, alcohol, oral contraceptive pill, smoking, some antibiotics, light, air, alkaline conditions.

VITAMINS
WATER-SOLUBLE

	RNI	FUNCTION
VITAMIN B12 COBALAMIN	Females and males 15+ years 1.5 mcg/day. No extra required during pregnancy. Lactation 2.0 mcg/day.	Forms and regenerates red blood cells, needed for DNA synthesis, maintains a healthy nervous system, needed for energy production.
FOLATE OR FOLIC ACID	Females and males 11+ years 200 mcg/day. Pregnancy 300 mcg/day (see also page 149). Lactation 260 mcg/day.	Works with B12 to protect and develop the nervous system and production of genetic material. Production of red blood cells for babies in utero. Protects against birth defects.
VITAMIN C ASCORBIC ACID	Females and males 15+ years 40 mg/day. Pregnancy 50 mg/day. Lactation 70 mg/day.	Collagen production, required for healthy, skin, bones, cartilage, teeth and blood vessels. Promotes healing, aids iron absorption. Also as a powerful antioxidant.
BIOTIN	No RNI. Intakes between 10 and 200 mcg/day are considered adequate and safe.	Essential for energy production and fat and protein metabolism. Needed for healthy skin and hair, and production of sex hormones.

OTHER WATER-SOLUBLE NUTRIENTS

FLAVONOIDS	No RNI.	Powerful antioxidants thought to reduce risk of chronic diseases like heart disease and cancer.
INOSITOL	No RNI. Can be made in the body from glucose.	Involved in relaying messages to the inside of cells. Combines with choline (see below) to form lecithin.
CHOLINE	No RNI. Can easily be made in the body.	Involved in cholesterol and fat metabolism, production of neuro-transmitters, promotes healthy cell membranes.

DEFICIENCY SIGNS	FOOD SOURCES	SYNERGISTS	ABSORPTION INHIBITORS
Pernicious anaemia, nerve problems.	Liver, heart, kidney, meat, poultry, fish, milk, cheese, eggs, fortified breakfast cereals.	Folate.	Exposure to air, light and vitamin C, antacids, laxatives, oral contraceptive pill, alcohol, anticonvulsants.
Anaemia, apathy, depression, swollen painful tongue, poor growth, problems with nerve development and functioning.	Dried yeast, liver, dark green leafy vegetables (eg. broccoli and cabbage), pulses, nuts, oat bran, yeast extract.	Other B vitamins especially B12 and B6, and vitamin C.	Exposure to air, light, heat and acidic conditions, alcohol, contraceptive pill, analgesics (aspirin), some antibiotics, anticonvulsants.
Loss of appetite, muscle cramps, dry skin, splitting hair, bleeding gums, bruising, nosebleeds, anaemia, infections, slow healing.	Citrus fruits, blackcurrants, strawberries, kiwi fruit, papaya, red chillies, broccoli, watercress, parsley, green leafy vegetables, red and green peppers.	Vitamin E, selenium.	Heat, light, oxygen, exposure to copper and iron cookware, bicarbonate of soda, contraceptive pill, anti-convulsants, analgesics.
Uncommon. Lethargy, nausea, thinning of hair, loss of hair colour, red skin rash, depression.	Brewer's yeast, liver, yeast extract, pulses, nuts, whole wheat, brown rice, milk, cheese, yoghurt, eggs.	Other B vitamins, sulphur.	Raw egg white, food processing, sulphur drugs. (Sulphur and biotin are synergists but they compete for absorption.)
Not known.	Most fruits and vegetables including citrus fruit (especially pith), buckwheat.	Vitamin C.	Water, cooking, heat, light, oxygen.
Raised cholesterol levels, nerve disorders, intestinal problems.	Wheat germ, cereals and pulses, oranges, peanuts.	Other B vitamins, choline.	Food processing, alcohol, coffee.
Rare. Unlikely in healthy people. Causes liver problems.	Eggs, egg yolks, liver, kidney, brain, lettuce, leafy green vegetables, wheat bran and germ, pulses.	Other B vitamins, inositol.	Food processing, alcohol.

MINERALS
MAJOR MINERALS

MAJOR MINERALS	RNI	FUNCTION
CALCIUM	Females and males 19+ years: 700 mg/day. No extra needed for pregnancy due to increased absorption. Lactation: 1250 mg/day.	Maintains strong bones and teeth, regulates nerve and muscle function, required for blood clotting and blood pressure regulation, enzyme regulation.
MAGNESIUM	Females 19+ years: 270 mg/day. No extra needed for pregnancy due to increased absorption. Lactation: 320 mg/day. Males 15+ years: 300 mg/day.	In combination with phosphorus and sodium, required for muscle and nerve function. Needed for energy. Maintains bone structure, regulates calcium balance.
PHOSPHORUS	Females and males 19+ years: 550 mg/day. No extra needed for pregnancy due to increased absorption. Lactation: 990 mg/day. Do not exceed 70 mg/kg body weight/day.	With calcium and magnesium, maintains bone structure. Needed for the production of energy in all body cells.
SODIUM	Females and males 15+ years: 1600 mg/day (equivalent to about 4g salt or sodium chloride). No extra needed for pregnancy or lactation. More than 3.2 g/day (about 8 g salt) may lead to raised blood pressure.	Works with potassium to regulate fluid and acid/alkali balance in the body and therefore responsible for nerve and muscle function.
POTASSIUM	Females and males 15+ years: 3500 mg/day. No extra needed for pregnancy or lactation.	Works with sodium to regulate the body's fluid balance, maintains normal blood pressure and heartbeat and nerve impulses.
CHLORIDE	Females and males 15+ years: 2500 mg/day. No extra needed for pregnancy or lactation.	Works with sodium and potassium to regulate acid/alkali and water balance.

DEFICIENCY SIGNS	FOOD SOURCES	SYNERGISTS	ABSORPTION INHIBITORS
Osteoporosis, osteomalacia, muscle spasms and cramping, rickets, high blood pressure, heart palpitations, joint pain.	Dairy products, canned fish eg. sardines and salmon eaten with their bones, some breakfast cereals, sesame seeds, almonds, green leafy vegetables, fortified soya milk and tofu.	Vitamin D, inositol, phosphorus, magnesium.	High phosphorus, salt or protein intake. Alcohol, oxalic acid (in chocolate, rhubarb), phytate eg. in bran, some laxatives, some diuretics, some antibiotics, large doses B complex pills.
Rare. Nausea, anxiety, muscle spasms, cramps, tremors, changes in blood pressure and heartbeat.	Nuts, soya beans, brewer's yeast, wholemeal bread and pasta, peas, seafood, dried fruit, seeds.	Calcium, vitamin D, phosphorus.	Alcohol, calcium carbonate antacid, some antibiotics, some diuretics.
Rare. Muscle weakness, bone pain, rickets, osteoporosis.	Meat, fish, dairy products, nuts, wheat bran, pumpkin, sunflower seeds, sesame seeds.	Calcium, magnesium, vitamin D.	Excess magnesium and aluminium.
Rare, can occur with chronic diarrhoea, vomiting, excess sweating.	Table salt, cured meats (eg. bacon), smoked fish, sauces, olives, canned food in brine, highly processed foods, cheese, butter, fatty snack foods, mineral waters.	Potassium, chloride.	Some diuretics, anti-gout drugs, some antibiotics, some laxatives.
Rare, can occur with chronic diarrhoea, vomiting, excess sweating. Confusion, cramps, fatigue, irregular heartbeat, extreme thirst.	Fresh fruit and vegetables (eg. apples, bananas, carrots, potatoes, broccoli, dates, oranges), wheat bran, fish, meat, poultry, milk and yoghurt.	Sodium, chloride.	Excess sodium, alcohol, coffee, some diuretics, some laxatives, some antibiotics, anti-gout drugs.
Rare.	Table salt, olives, tomato sauce, bacon, canned fish, cheese, peanuts, processed foods containing salt.	Sodium, potassium.	Not applicable.

MINERALS
MAJOR MINERALS

	RNI	FUNCTION
SULPHUR S	No RNI. Most comes from the proteins we eat.	Essential for healthy hair, skin and nails. Needed for protein synthesis and for detoxifying drugs and protecting cells from oxidative damage.

MINERALS
TRACE MINERALS

IRON Fe	Females 11–50 years: 14.8 mg/day. Females 50+ years: 8.7mg/day. Males 19+ years: 8.7 mg/day. No extra usually needed for pregnancy or lactation.	Oxygen transport and storage in muscles, improves immunity, required for growth, energy production, drug metabolism and proper mental functioning.
ZINC Zn	Females 15+ years: 7 mg/day. No extra required during pregnancy. Lactation: 0–4 months 13 mg/day. 4+ months 9.5 mg/day. Male 15+ years: 9.5 mg/day. Acute intake of 2 g zinc produces nausea. Regularly consuming more than 50 mg/day may interfere with copper metabolism.	Improves immunity, healing. Needed for healthy eyes, skin, nails, for growth and sexual development, for the activity of enzymes, for DNA and protein synthesis, and activity of vitamins A and D.
COPPER Cu	Females and males 19+ years: 1.2 mg/day. No extra needed during pregnancy. Lactation: 1.5 mg/day. High intakes are harmful. In some countries, levels of 1.6 mg per litre in drinking water have been associated with toxic effects.	Needed for iron and fat metabolism, connective tissue synthesis, maintenance of the heart muscle, functioning of the nervous and immune systems, maintains red blood cell membranes.

DEFICIENCY SIGNS	FOOD SOURCES	SYNERGISTS	ABSORPTION INHIBITORS
Rare. Usually only occurs with a diet that is very low in protein.	Eggs, meat, chicken, fish, seafood, kidney, heart, liver, spinach, nuts, Brussels sprouts, bread, cheese, dried fruits.	Thiamin, biotin.	Not applicable.
Anaemia, reduced physical and mental performance, fatigue, poor circulation, depression, decreased resistance to infection and illness.	Red meat, liver, clams, mussels, oysters, chicken, fish, eggs, spinach and other green leafy vegetables, dried apricots, cocoa powder, fortified breakfast cereals, wholemeal bread.	Vitamin C.	Phytate (seeds, nuts, grains), large quantities tea/coffee, calcium supplements, analgesics (aspirin), narcotics (codeine, morphine), some antacids, some antibiotics and anti-gout drugs.
White spots on nails, loss of taste and appetite, poor growth and wound healing, night blindness, late onset of puberty, dry flaky skin, dandruff, increased susceptibility to infection.	Oysters, crab and shellfish, other seafood, red meat, chicken, liver, kidney, dairy products, some green vegetables, eggs, nuts and wheat germ.	Vitamin A, vitamin D, copper.	Alcohol, some diuretics, some drugs, oral contraceptive pill, hormone replacement therapy, phytate (seeds, nuts, grains), large amounts of tea, coffee, diet high in iron, iron supplements.
Uncommon. Anaemia, decreased immunity, blood vessel and bone weakening, red blood cell damage, arthritis, impaired growth, and heart muscle and nervous system degeneration.	Shellfish (oysters, lobster, crab), offal (eg. liver), nuts and seeds, wholegrains, prunes, soya products.	Zinc, iron.	High zinc diet. Zinc supplements. High intake of iron. (Copper, zinc and iron are synergists, but compete for absorption.) High intake of manganese, molybdenum, vitamin C and antacids.

MINERALS
TRACE MINERALS

	RNI	FUNCTION
MANGANESE	Safe intake: Adults more than 1.4 mg/day.	Functions together with zinc and copper in a major antioxidant compound. Involved in carbohydrate and fat metabolism and brain function.
IODINE	Females and males 15+ years: 140 mcg/day. No extra needed for pregnancy or lactation. Do not exceed 17 mcg/kg/day (or 1000 mcg/day). Excessively high intake may cause hyperthyroidism.	Essential component of the thyroid hormones which regulate metabolic rate, growth and development, and promote protein synthesis.
CHROMIUM	Safe intake:. Adults more than 25 mcg/day.	Needed for insulin to function normally and for glucose to enter cells. Involved in fat and protein metabolism.
MOLYBDENUM	Safe intake: Adults 50–400 mcg/day.	Required for enzymes involved in producing waste products before they are excreted (detoxification), and oxidation and detoxification of many other compounds.
FLUORIDE	No RNI or safe intake for adults.	Prevents tooth decay and discolouration, strengthens bones.
SELENIUM	Females 15+ years: 60 mcg/day. No extra needed for pregnancy. Lactation: 75 mcg/day. Males 19+ years: 75 mcg/day.	Works with vitamin E in an antioxidant enzyme. Needed for synthesis of thyroid hormones which regulate basal metabolic rate.

DEFICIENCY SIGNS	FOOD SOURCES	SYNERGISTS	ABSORPTION INHIBITORS
Rare. Growth retardation, bone abnormalities, brain and reproductive function problems, fat and carbohydrate metabolism problems.	Nuts, sesame seeds, wheat germ, wheat bran, oat bran, legumes, blackberries, spinach.	Copper, zinc.	Not applicable.
Goitre (enlarged thyroid gland, swelling in the neck), metabolic rate drops, bulging eyes, fatigue, mental retardation, hair loss, slow reflexes, dry skin.	Iodised salt, seafood (eg. clams, haddock, oysters, salmon, sardines), dairy products, eggs, seaweed.	Selenium.	Goitrogen substances in foods (turnips, cabbage, cassava, Brussels sprouts).
High blood glucose and insulin levels. High blood cholesterol and triglyceride levels.	Egg yolk, red meat, liver, dairy products, whole grains, nuts, potato, oysters, clams, rye bread, wine, chillies, spinach, oranges, apple peel, wholegrain bread.		Not applicable.
Rare, only seen in hospital patients on deficient feed tubes. Impaired growth, reduced appetite.	Grains, legumes, dairy products, spinach, cauliflower, peas, corn, kidneys, liver.		Not applicable.
Increased tooth decay, particularly up to the age of 13 years.	Fluoridated water, tea, fish eaten with bones, milk, Cheddar cheese. Also fluoridated toothpaste.	Calcium.	Aluminium cookware.
Seen in areas with low selenium soil levels. Muscular aches and weakness. A form of heart disease called Keshan disease.	Seafood, liver, kidney, eggs, meat, wholegrains, brazil nuts, wheat germ, wholegrain bread.	Vitamin E, iodine.	Not applicable.

VITAMINS AND OTHER NUTRIENTS

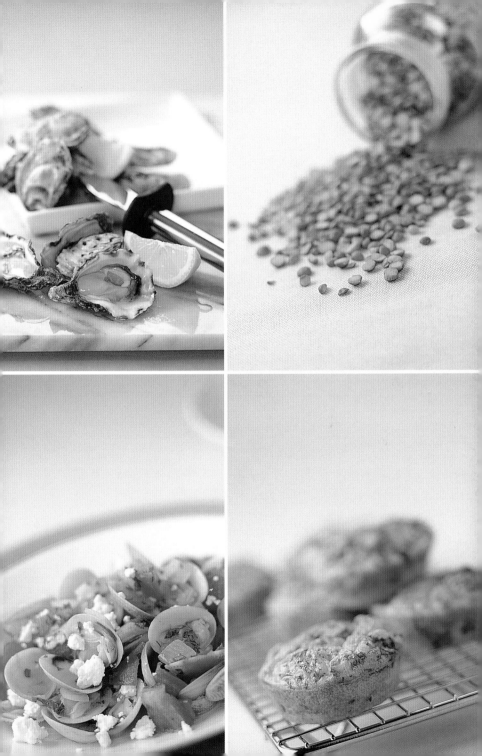

VITAMINS – FAT-SOLUBLE
VITAMIN A

REFERENCE NUTRIENT INTAKE
Men: 700 mcg RE^{+}/day Women: 600 mcg RE/day
($^{+}$ RE see page 112)

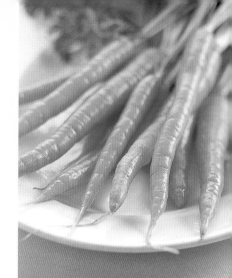

FOOD SOURCES	mcg RE per 100 g
Liver, calf, fried	25200
Liver, lamb, fried	19700
Liver, chicken, fried	10500
Pâté, liver	7400
Carrots, raw	1353
Carrots, boiled	1260
Low fat spread	1084
Margarine	905
Butter	887
Sweet potato, baked	855
Red chillies	685
Parsley	673
Double cream	654
Red peppers (capsicum)	640
Spinach, boiled	640
Butternut squash, baked	548
Cream cheese	422
Watercress	420
Mixed frozen vegetables, boiled	420
Spring greens, boiled	378
Hard cheese	373
Tomatoes, grilled	307
Mangoes	300
Chicken eggs, whole, cooked or raw	190
Papaya (Pawpaw)	165
Canteloupe melon	165
Greek yoghurt	121
Tomatoes	107
Apricots, dried	105
Broccoli, boiled	80
Milk, whole	56

Vitamin A is essential for good vision, hence the belief that carrots are good for your eyesight. Vitamin A requirement may be increased if you strain your eyes watching too much television, working in poor light or glare, or looking at a computer screen all day.

RECIPE Combine slices of a fresh ripe mango, chunks of canteloupe melon, some finely shredded ginger, chopped dried apricots, hazelnuts and sprigs of fresh mint. Drizzle with a little lime juice and sprinkle with cinnamon. This is a great way to start the day with vitamin A.

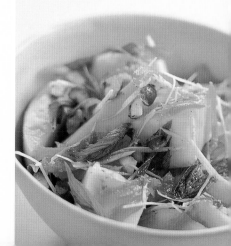

RECIPE Marinate chicken livers in a Japanese-style teriyaki marinade, then thread them onto skewers and barbecue or grill them.

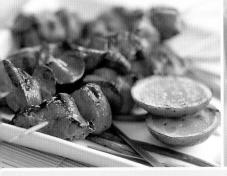

A glass of carrot and ginger juice is an excellent source of carotenoids for those who eat breakfast on the run.

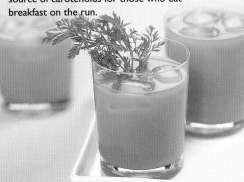

VITAMIN A is a fat-soluble vitamin and comes in two forms:

PREFORMED VITAMIN A (retinoids) that we obtain from foods of animal origin, such as liver and dairy products.

PROVITAMIN A (beta- carotene and other carotenoids) which can be converted to active vitamin A in the body, and comes from red and yellow fruits, dark green leafy vegetables, and vegetables such as carrots (from which they derive their name).

Vitamin A is essential for good vision, assists the growth and repair of body tissues and helps maintain soft skin and hair. Beta carotene is a powerful antioxidant vitamin.

Approximately one third of the carotene in food is converted to vitamin A. Light cooking, puréeing and mashing ruptures the cell membrane and makes the carotene more readily available.

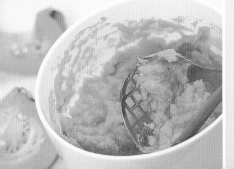

CAUTION Vitamin A can build up to toxic levels. Don't exceed 9000 mcg RE/day (men); 7500 mcg RE/day (women). Vitamin A supplements (including any fish oil supplements high in vitamin A) should be avoided by pregnant women and people who are taking vitamin A acne preparations or broad-spectrum antibiotics. Food is the best source of vitamin A because high-dose supplements containing 4–10 times the RNI can cause birth defects and health problems.

VITAMINS — FAT-SOLUBLE
VITAMIN D

REFERENCE NUTRIENT INTAKE
No RNI because vitamin D can be made in the skin. Except men and women 65+ years: 10 mcg/day. Pregnancy and lactation 10 mcg/day.

FOOD SOURCES	mcg per 100 g
Cod liver oil	210
Kippers, baked	25
Salmon, red, canned in brine	23
Herring, grilled	16.1
Pilchards, canned in tomato sauce	14
Sardines, grilled	12.3
Trout, grilled	11
Salmon, grilled	9.6
Smoked mackerel	8
Low-fat spread and margarines	8
Mackerel, grilled	5.4
Egg yolk	4.9
Sardines, canned in brine	4.6
Tuna, canned in brine	4.0
Evaporated milk	4.0
Fortified breakfast cereals	2.7
Scrambled egg with milk	1.9
Eggs, whole	1.8
Butter	0.8
Beef, lamb, pork, chicken	0.3–0.8
Cheddar cheese	0.3
Yoghurt, whole milk, plain	0.04
Milk, whole	0.03
White fish	Traces
Crustaceans/molluscs	Traces

People with dark skin require less vitamin D than those with fairer skin. Sunscreens with factor 8 or higher actually prohibit the synthesis of vitamin D, but most people get enough sunshine to compensate. Smoke, pollution, window glass and clothing can block sunlight and therefore reduce vitamin D synthesis.

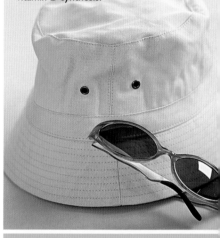

We don't rely on our diet for vitamin D because most of us make enough in our bodies after being in the sun. However, eating sardines is a delicious way to incorporate small amounts of this vitamin and other essential nutrients into our diet.

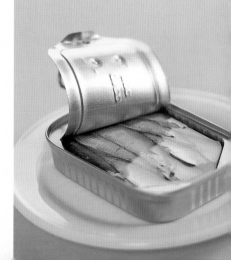

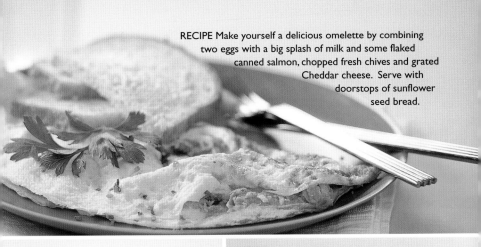

RECIPE Make yourself a delicious omelette by combining two eggs with a big splash of milk and some flaked canned salmon, chopped fresh chives and grated Cheddar cheese. Serve with doorstops of sunflower seed bread.

Children need more vitamin D than adults. Without it their bones and teeth will not develop and harden. Adequate sunshine and eating plenty of dairy products regularly throughout life will help keep bones strong.

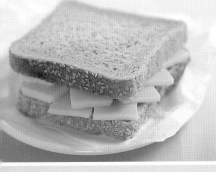

Full-fat milk contains some vitamin D, although skimmed milk contains only traces. Fortified milks are sometimes available, which have added vitamin D.

VITAMIN D is a fat-soluble vitamin. It

is known as the sunshine vitamin because it can be made in the skin when the skin is exposed to ultraviolet light. In summer, two hours of sunlight each week is sufficient to maintain adequate levels. Once made, vitamin D is stored in the body for use over the winter, so most people do not have to rely on diet. It is needed for calcium and phosphorus absorption and healthy bones and teeth.

DEFICIENCY Some people who don't get enough sunlight or vitamin D in their diet are at risk of developing osteomalacia – a condition causing the bones to become soft and easily broken. For more information see page 167. For children, prolonged deficiency may result in rickets, a bone disorder characterised by soft bones, bow legs and curvature of the spine. Vitamin D supplements are advisable for people at risk of osteomalacia.

TOXICITY Too much vitamin D from fortified foods and supplements (more than 50 mcg a day) can be toxic. Effects include sore eyes, itchy skin, vomiting, kidney and heart damage.

VITAMINS – FAT-SOLUBLE

VITAMIN E

SAFE INTAKE:
Men: above 4 mg/day.
Women: above 3 mg/day.

FOOD SOURCES	mg per 100 g
Wheat germ oil	137
Sunflower oil	49.2
Safflower oil	40.7
Sunflower seeds	37.8
Palm oil	33.1
Polyunsaturated margarine	32.6
Hazelnuts	25
Almonds	24
Tomatoes, sun-dried	24
Rapeseed oil	22.2
Wheat germ	22
Mayonnaise	19
Soya oil	16.1
Peanut oil	15.2
Pine nuts	13.6
Salad cream	10.6
Peanuts	10.1
Brazil nuts	7.2
Low-fat spread	6.3
Peanut butter	5
Bombay mix	4.7
Tomatoes, grilled	4
Walnuts	3.8
Pesto sauce	3.8
Avocado	3.2
Sesame seeds	2.5
Butter	2.0
Spinach	1.7
Salmon, pink, canned in brine	1.5
Eggs, raw, boiled or poached	1.1
Broccoli, boiled	1.1
Cheese, Parmesan	0.7

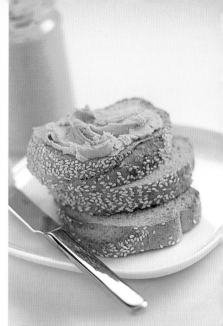

Thick slices of wholegrain bread topped with peanut butter is a great lunch to have to help your vitamin E intake.

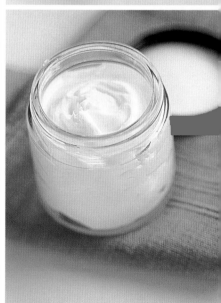

Applied topically in the form of vitamin E cream, the vitamin is absorbed through the skin and promotes wound healing.

Vitamin E is destroyed by heat and exposure to light. Although it's relatively stable at normal cooking temperatures, the high temperatures used in deep-frying, and the repeated heating of the oil, tend to destroy most of the vitamin E. The best way to get this vitamin from oils is in salad dressings.

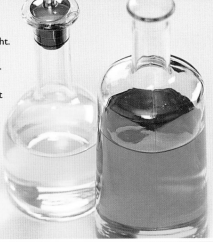

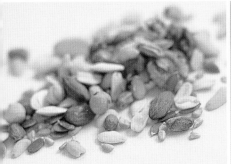

There are eight naturally occurring forms of vitamin E, the most common being alpha-tocopherol. Include plenty of the good sources, such as nuts, plant oils, and wheat germ in your diet.

VITAMIN E is a fat-soluble vitamin and a very powerful antioxidant that neutralises free radical compounds before they can damage cell membranes. It helps protect us from the damage caused by pollution and heavy metals. It is essential for healing, prevention of scarring, and healthy red blood cells and nerves. Deficiency is relatively rare because it is found in many foods.

RECIPE Cook pasta and toss with a kind of pesto made using fresh rocket, almonds, grated Parmesan cheese and oil.

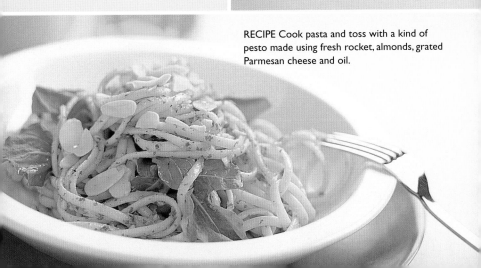

VITAMIN K

SAFE INTAKE
Adults 1 mcg per kg body weight/day.

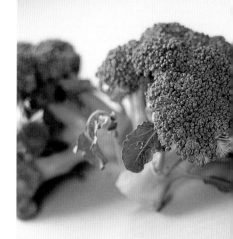

FOOD SOURCES	mcg per 100 g*
Spinach	240
Lettuce	200
Soya beans	190
Cauliflower	150
Cabbage	100
Broccoli	100
Wheat bran	80
Wheat germ	37
Green beans	22
Asparagus	21
Oats	20
Potatoes	20
Peas	19
Strawberries	13
Pork	11
Beef mince	7
Milk, full cream	5
Milk, skimmed	4

To retain the vitamins in your vegetables, don't cook them too long, but just until they are tender. To prevent vitamin K deficiency, eat plenty of the vegetables listed, including delicious broccoli.

Vitamin K is probably best known for its role in promoting blood clotting to stop bleeding. Because of this, the vitamin is often referred to as the band-aid vitamin.

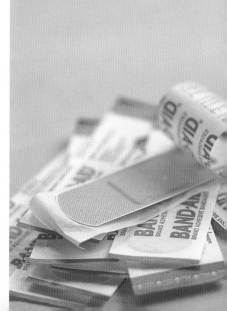

*Australian values.

Eating bio yoghurts (containing acidophilus bacteria) will help you maintain your levels of intestinal bacteria and therefore ensure you make vitamin K in your body. This is particularly useful if you are taking a course of antibiotics, some of which inhibit absorption of the vitamin.

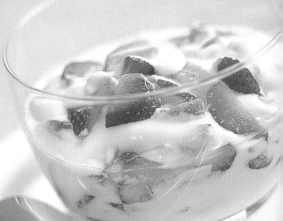

RECIPE Stir-fry sliced pork fillet with broccoli florets, sliced mushrooms, shelled peas, sliced beans, roughly chopped spinach and a little soy sauce and honey.

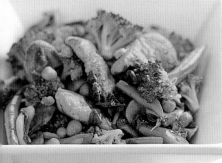

Breakfast is a good time to include vitamin K in your diet with plenty of oats, wheat bran, wheat germ and milk.

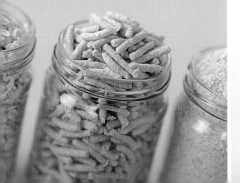

VITAMIN K is a fat-soluble vitamin available in a limited number of foods and also made in the body by bacteria which live in our intestinal tract. Babies are given an injection of vitamin K at birth because the infant gut is free of bacteria and breast milk does not contain much of the vitamin. Vitamin K promotes blood clotting and is required for bone mineralisation and kidney function.

DEFICIENCY This is very rare in healthy people but can result from long-term antibiotic use. Newborn babies are at risk, as explained above, and are therefore injected with the vitamin. Signs of deficiency are easy bruising, and uncontrolled bleeding after injury and surgery.

TOXICITY It is hard to get too much vitamin K from foods, but high doses of supplements containing vitamin K can be dangerous, especially if you are taking anticoagulant drugs. Large doses may also cause flushing and sweating.

ESSENTIAL FATTY ACIDS

No RNI. Suggest approximately 1 per cent of total energy intake.

SOURCES OF OMEGA-3 FATTY ACIDS

Anchovies, canned, fresh

Canola oil

Cod liver oil

Egg yolk (chicken and duck)

Flaxseed oil

Hazelnuts

Mackerel, canned, fresh

Oysters

Pecans

Prawns

Salmon (pink and red), canned, fresh

Sardines, canned, fresh

Soya bean oil

Squid

Sunflower oil

Tuna, fresh

Vegetables, green leafy

Walnuts

SOURCES OF OMEGA-6 FATTY ACIDS

Canola oil

Corn oil

Dairy and oil spreads

Evening primrose oil

Flaxseed oil

Nuts

Olive oil

Safflower oil

Soya beans

Sunflower oil

If enough omega-3 fatty acids are consumed in the diet, other important fatty acids can be synthesised in the body. Oily fish with dark flesh, such as mackerel, tuna, salmon and sardines, are the most concentrated source of omega-3 fatty acids. Aim for two or more portions of fish every week, one of which should be an oily fish.

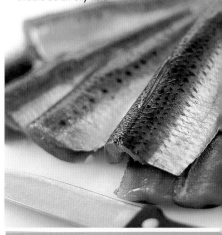

Like other polyunsaturated fats, essential fatty acids may help control blood cholesterol levels and reduce the risk of heart disease when eaten in place of saturated fats in a low-fat diet.

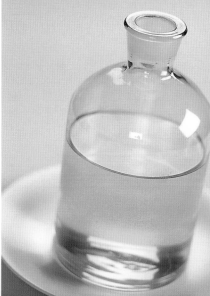

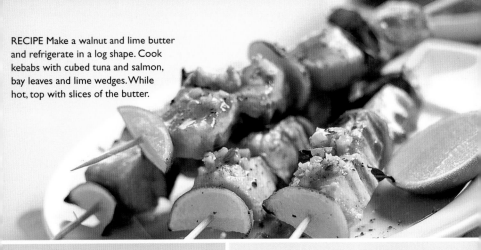

RECIPE Make a walnut and lime butter and refrigerate in a log shape. Cook kebabs with cubed tuna and salmon, bay leaves and lime wedges. While hot, top with slices of the butter.

Essential fatty acids must be supplied by the diet. If fish is not your thing, then walnuts, pecans, soya beans and tahini are good sources. Canned soya beans make a tasty houmous.

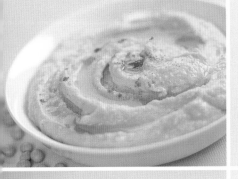

ESSENTIAL FATTY ACIDS are

fatty acids that can't be made in the body and must be consumed in the diet. Linoleic acid (omega-6) and alpha-linolenic acid (omega-3) are the essential fatty acids and are important for growth, healthy skin and the proper function of eyes and nerves. Linoleic acid and alpha-linolenic acid can be used by the body to make other types of fatty acids.

Cold-pressed vegetable oils, especially sunflower, corn, soya bean, sesame and safflower, are high in omega-6 fatty acids. A balance of both omega-3 and omega-6 is vital and this can be achieved by a mixture of flaxseed oil with the above oils. Canola oil has the best ratio of both omega-3 and omega-6 fatty acids, and soya and walnut oil also contain a mix of both.

DEFICIENCY If essential fatty acids aren't consumed in sufficient amounts, a deficiency results. Symptoms include scaly, dry skin, poor healing of wounds, liver problems, growth failure in infants and impaired vision and hearing.

PROTECTION Although omega-3 fatty acids do not affect cholesterol levels in the blood, they do reduce the tendency for the blood to clot, thereby reducing the risk of heart disease.

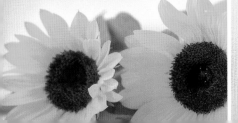

VITAMINS – WATER-SOLUBLE

VITAMIN B1 (THIAMIN)

REFERENCE NUTRIENT INTAKE
Women: 0.8 mg/day (Pregnancy: 0.9 mg/day.
Lactation: 1.0 mg/day). Men 19–50 years: 1.0 mg/day.
Men 51+ years: 0.9 mg/day.

FOOD SOURCES	mg per 100 g
Quorn myco-protein	37
Meat extract	9.7
Yeast extract	4.1
Wheat germ	2
Fortified breakfast cereals	1.03–1.8
Sunflower seeds	1.6
Pork fillet, lean, grilled	1.6
Bacon, back, grilled	1.2
Gammon rashers, grilled	1.2
Peanuts, plain	1.1
Malted milk powder	1.0
Tahini	0.9
Wheat bran	0.9
Sesame seeds	0.9
Ham, lean	0.8
Soya flour	0.8
Peas, boiled	0.7
Pine nuts	0.7
Pistachio nuts, roasted and salted	0.7
Cashew nuts	0.7
Liver, chicken and calf, fried	0.6
Wheat germ	0.5
Kidney, lamb	0.3
Wholemeal bread	0.3
Pasta, wholemeal, boiled	0.2
Kidney beans, canned	0.2
Red split lentils, boiled	0.2
Rice, brown, boiled	0.1
Soya beans, boiled	0.1

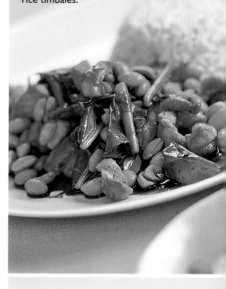

RECIPE Stir-fry strips of pork fillet with Chinese leaf, roasted peanuts and soya beans in a little peanut oil. Add soya sauce or oyster sauce. Serve with brown or wild rice timbales.

Absorption of thiamin is increased in the presence of allinin, a substance which naturally occurs in garlic and onions.

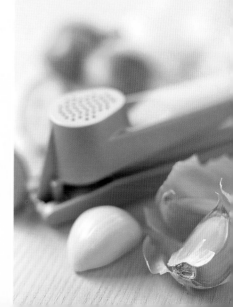

Thiamin occurs in limited quantities in most foods but is available in large quantities in pork and offal.

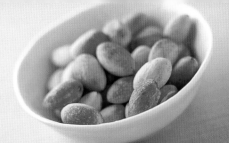

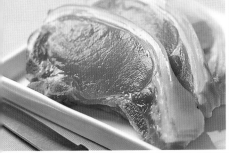

Many nuts, as well as sunflower seeds, will assist in adding thiamin to your diet. However, foods containing sulphur dioxide, such as wine and dried fruits, and sulphite, used in the making of sausages and bacon, can inhibit thiamin absorption.

VITAMIN B1 (THIAMIN) is a water-soluble vitamin. It is essential for the nervous system and DNA synthesis. Along with other B vitamins, it is needed by the body to produce energy from the nutrients carbohydrate, protein and fat. It is also necessary for growth in childhood and fertility in adults.

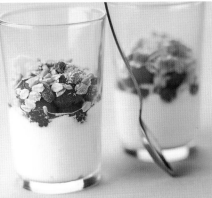

RECIPE For breakfast, layer in a glass some yoghurt, fresh fruit, muesli, oat bran, wheat germ, sunflower and sesame seeds.

Thiamin is found in the germ and bran of wheat and the husk of rice, so consumption of wholegrain bread will provide thiamin in the diet.

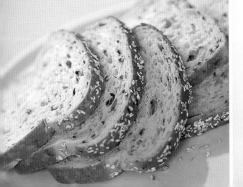

DEFICIENCY Thiamin deficiency is rare but can occur in chronic alcoholics. Extreme deficiency results in the disease beri-beri. Early deficiency symptoms include nausea, muscle fatigue, cramps, depression, irritability and poor coordination. Supplements with relatively large doses of thiamin (50 mg) are marketed for stress relief or an energy boost, but, unless a person has a deficiency, these won't help relieve stress or tiredness. Thiamin absorption is inhibited by an enzyme (thiaminase) present in raw fish and shellfish. Thiamin levels can also be depleted during food preparation, cooking or storage because thiamin is sensitive to heat and oxygen.

VITAMIN B2 (RIBOFLAVIN)

REFERENCE NUTRIENT INTAKE
Women: 1.1 mg/day. (Pregnancy: 1.4 mg/day
Lactation: 1.6 mg/day).
Men: 1.3 mg/day.

FOOD SOURCES	mg per 100 g
Yeast extract	11.9
Meat extract	8.5
Liver, lamb, fried	5.7
Kidney, pig, fried	3.7
Liver, chicken, fried	2.7
Fortified breakfast cereals	1.0–2.2
Malted milk powder	1.3
Pate, liver	1.2
Almonds	0.8
Wheat germ	0.8
Goat's milk soft cheese	0.6
Muesli, swiss-style	0.7
Hard cheese	0.4–0.5
Egg yolk	0.5
Goose or duck, roasted	0.5
Smoked mackerel	0.5
Tomato-based pasta sauce	0.5
Chocolate, milk	0.5
Tempeh	0.5
Cheese, brie	0.4
Cheese, stilton	0.4
Evaporated milk	0.4
Fromage frais, plain	0.4
Wheat bran	0.4
Eggs, boiled	0.4
Mushrooms, raw	0.3
Pilchards or sardines, canned, in tomato sauce	0.3
Ham hock	0.2
Split peas, boiled	0.06
Kale, boiled	0.06
Spinach, boiled	0.05

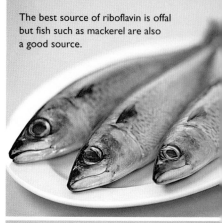

The best source of riboflavin is offal but fish such as mackerel are also a good source.

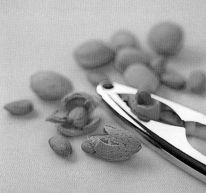

Almonds are a great source of riboflavin. They are a simple snack and easy to add to muesli, salads and stir-fries.

Top up your riboflavin intake first thing in the morning. A breakfast of muesli, a hard-boiled egg and toast with yeast extract is ideal.

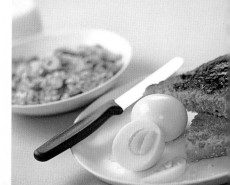

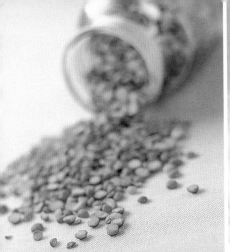

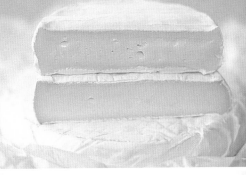

A moderate amount of riboflavin is contained in a variety of cheeses.

Keep up your riboflavin levels by regularly eating foods containing riboflavin. A simple way of adding a small amount of riboflavin to your diet is to make a delicious split pea soup, using ham hock for flavour. Riboflavin forms part of enzymes which are involved in energy metabolism so you may need more when you are using a lot of energy.

RECIPE Whip up mini mushroom frittatas. Whisk together three eggs, add a generous splash of milk and some chopped fresh flat-leaf parsley and grated Parmesan. Fry some sliced mushrooms and spring onions in butter and add to the eggs. Bake in muffin tins.

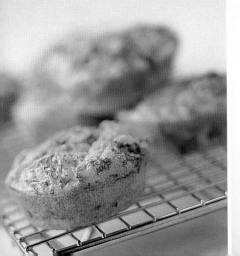

VITAMIN B2 (RIBOFLAVIN) is a water-soluble vitamin essential for producing energy from carbohydrate, protein and fat. It is necessary for healthy skin, hair and nails, and good vision. It is involved in converting other vitamins (K, B3, B6 and folate) into their active forms in the body. Unlike many vitamins, riboflavin is stable in the presence of heat and acid, but is destroyed by alkali and light.

DEFICIENCY Riboflavin deficiency usually occurs in conjunction with deficiencies in other B vitamins. Deficiency signs are quite obvious, the most common being cracks in the sides of the mouth, a red, sore tongue, or a feeling you have sand in your eyes, which can also be watery or bloodshot. Skin problems are also a sign, especially scaly, flaky dermatitis around the nose and ears. As with thiamin, riboflavin supplements are promoted for an energy boost, but they are not likely to produce any benefits unless a person is truly deficient. Improving your diet gives you more health benefits.

VITAMIN B3 (NIACIN)

REFERENCE NUTRIENT INTAKE

Women 19–50 years: 13 mg NE⁺/day. Women 51+ years:
12 mg NE/day. (Lactation: 15 mg NE/day.) Men 19–50 years: 17 mg
NE/day. Men 51+ years: 16 mg NE/day. (⁺ NE see page 10.)

FOOD SOURCES	mg per 100 g
Yeast extract	73
Wheat bran	32.6
Liver, lamb, fried	24.8
Tuna, canned in oil	21.1
Fortified breakfast cereals	10–21
Turkey, light meat, roasted	19.7
Peanut butter	19
Liver, calf, fried	19.4
Peanuts, plain	19.3
Chicken, light meat, roasted	18.1
Malted milk powder	17.4
Liver, chicken, fried	17.3
Nuts, mixed	14.8
Mackerel, smoked	13
Beef, fillet, lean, grilled	12.9
Salmon, grilled	12.2
Bacon, back, grilled	11
Sesame seeds	10.4
Salmon, pink, canned in brine	10.3
Tahini	9.2
Sunflower seeds	9.1
Anchovy, canned in oil	8.5
Trout, rainbow, grilled	8.2
Almonds	6.5
Cashew nuts, roasted, salted	6.5
Cheese, Cheddar	6.1
Wholemeal bread	5.9
Eggs, boiled or raw	3.8
Pasta, wholemeal, boiled	2.3
Rice, brown, boiled	1.9
Potatoes, baked	1.1
Milk, whole	0.8

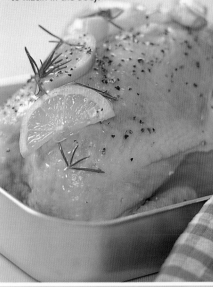

Eating foods such as chicken, fish and nuts,
which contain tryptophan, will ensure higher
levels of niacin because tryptophan converts
to niacin in the body.

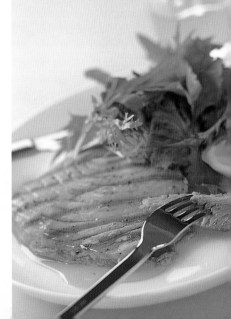

Tuna, trout, salmon, halibut, mackerel and
swordfish all contain generous quantities
of niacin.

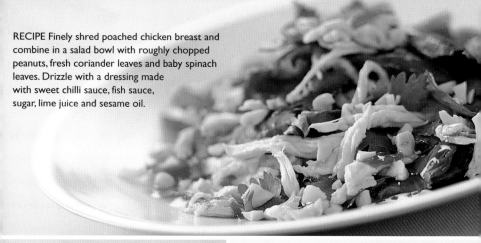

RECIPE Finely shred poached chicken breast and combine in a salad bowl with roughly chopped peanuts, fresh coriander leaves and baby spinach leaves. Drizzle with a dressing made with sweet chilli sauce, fish sauce, sugar, lime juice and sesame oil.

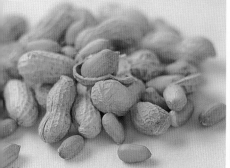

Nuts are a nutritious snack or addition to meals and are a good way of ensuring there is niacin in your diet.

VITAMIN B3 (NIACIN) is an

extremely stable water-soluble vitamin and isn't really affected by light, heat, acid, alkali or air. It can be made in the body through the conversion of the amino acid tryptophan. Niacin is important for the production of energy from carbohydrate, protein and fat. It is necessary for healthy skin, tongue and digestive tissues, as well as for normal mental functioning.

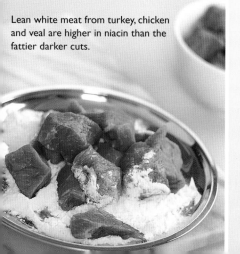

Lean white meat from turkey, chicken and veal are higher in niacin than the fattier darker cuts.

DEFICIENCY Severe deficiency causes pellagra. It is rare in western countries but occurs in countries with food shortages and diets low in protein. A lack of niacin may lead to minor skin problems, weakness, general fatigue and loss of appetite.

TOXICITY If you buy niacin supplements, make sure you buy the nicotinamide form normally sold in the UK. Niacin in the form of nicotinic acid should only be taken on medical advice. Often prescribed to help decrease cholesterol and triglyceride levels, nicotinic acid has the side effect of relaxing blood vessels, causing flushing, red skin rash, high blood sugar levels, itching and even fainting.

VITAMIN B5 (PANTOTHENIC ACID)

No RNI. Intakes of 3–7 mg/day are considered adequate.

FOOD SOURCES	mg per 100 g
Dried yeast	11
Liver, lamb, fried	8.0
Broad beans, canned	6.7
Liver, chicken, fried	5.9
Egg yolk, raw	4.6
Kidney, lamb, fried	4.6
Liver, calf, fried	4.1
Pork fillet, lean, grilled	2.2
Peanuts, plain	2.7
Wheat bran	2.4
Sesame seeds	2.1
Mushrooms, raw	2.0
Salmon, steamed	1.8
Pecan nuts	1.7
Peanut butter	1.7
Soya flour	1.6
Trout, rainbow, grilled	1.6
Chicken breast, grilled, no skin	1.6
Walnuts	1.6
Hazelnuts	1.5
Duck, roast	1.5
Eggs, boiled or poached	1.3
Avocado	1.1
Cashew nuts	1.1
Ham, lean	1.0
Lobster, boiled	1.0
Dried dates	0.8
Dried apricots	0.7
Wholemeal bread	0.6
Cheese, Danish, blue	0.5
Yoghurt, whole, plain	0.5

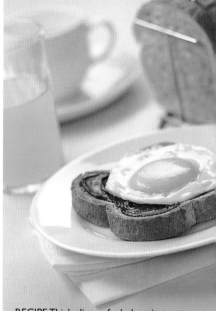

RECIPE Thick slices of wholegrain toast spread with yeast extract and topped with a poached or fried egg.

Pantothenic acid is particularly abundant in animal products including meat, offal, dairy products and eggs. Foods containing moulds, such as mould-ripened cheeses and yoghurts, and yeasts are high in vitamin B5.

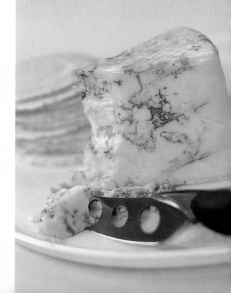

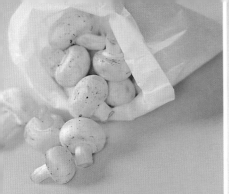

All mushrooms contain a generous amount of vitamin B5, but frying will reduce the vitamins so it is better to eat them raw.

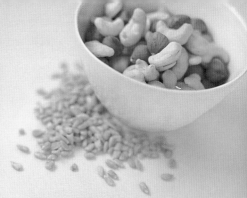

Eating a variety of nuts and seeds is an easy way to top up your B5 intake.

RECIPE Fresh mushroom caps drizzled with melted parsley butter and finished with crumbled blue cheese, then sprinkled with sesame seeds and grilled.

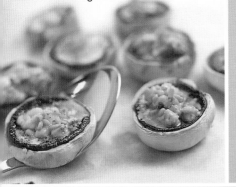

VITAMIN B5 (PANTOTHENIC ACID) is a water-soluble vitamin required for the reactions involved in protein, fat and carbohydrate metabolism. It is needed for fatty acid, cholesterol and steroid hormone synthesis. This vitamin occurs in a wide variety of foods, so deficiency is rare but may be seen with other B vitamin deficiencies, resulting from chronic alcoholism or malnutrition.

Vitamin B5 is depleted through processing and when foods are cooked with acids (vinegars, citrus) and alkali (baking soda). Dry heat cooking methods (frying, grilling) are more damaging to the vitamin than moist heat methods such as stewing and poaching.

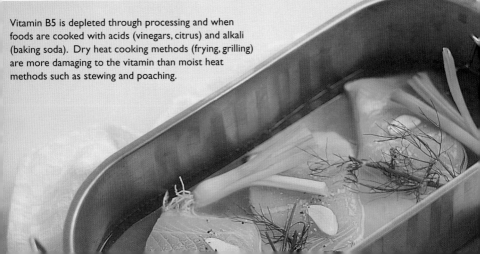

VITAMINS – WATER-SOLUBLE
VITAMIN B6 (PYRIDOXINE)

RECOMMENDED DAILY INTAKE
Men 1.3–1.9 mg Women 0.9– 1.4 mg
Pregnant 1–1.5 mg Lactating 1.6–2.2 mg

FOOD SOURCES	mg per 100 grams
VEGEMITE (YEAST EXTRACT)	3
DRIED YEAST	2
WHEAT BRAN	1.4
OATMEAL, COOKED	1.4
WHEAT GERM	1.3
GARLIC	1.2
SESAME SEEDS	0.79
SUNFLOWER SEEDS	0.77
WALNUTS	0.7
MACKEREL, FRESH	0.66
SALMON, FRESH	0.65
SOY FLOUR	0.65
CHICKEN LIVER	0.58
HAZELNUTS	0.56
TUNA, FRESH	0.53
BEEF KIDNEY	0.52
BANANAS	0.51
PEANUT BUTTER	0.5
SALMON, PINK, CANNED	0.5
WHOLEMEAL FLOUR	0.5
CALVES' LIVER	0.49
SNAPPER	0.46
PORK, LEAN	0.45
AVOCADO	0.42
FETA CHEESE	0.42
HALIBUT	0.4
SARDINES, CANNED	0.4
TUNA, CANNED	0.4
BEEF, LEAN	0.38

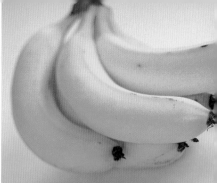

Vitamin B6 is found in a wide variety of plant and animal foods and is added to some breakfast cereals. Boost your levels by adding bananas to your daily diet.

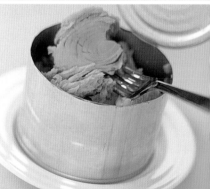

Oily fish, as well as prawns, are high in vitamin B6. A 200 g serve of tuna, salmon or mackerel will provide your daily requirement of this vitamin.

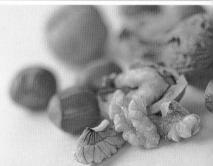

Snacking on unsalted mixed nuts is a good way to get your daily intake of vitamin B6. Eating a cupful of mixed nuts will give you enough B6 for one day.

RECIPE Make a breakfast smoothie that has lots of vitamin B6. Blend soy milk, yoghurt, banana, hazelnuts, wheat germ and maple syrup. Team it with a couple of slices of toasted wholegrain bread topped with sliced tomato and avocado, a drizzle of lime juice and plenty of cracked pepper.

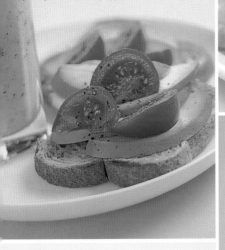

Sashimi salmon is a great way to get B6 into your diet. Thinly slice top-quality boneless salmon fillets and serve with a little soy sauce and wasabi.

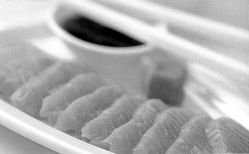

VITAMIN B6 (PYRIDOXINE) is

a water-soluble vitamin that is essential for releasing energy from amino acids (protein) and for the metabolism of fat and carbohydrate. It is also required for the normal functioning of the nervous system, as well as the formation of haemoglobin and white cells, and therefore for the immune system.

RECIPE Make wholemeal banana muffins, adding wheat bran and chopped walnuts to the mixture.

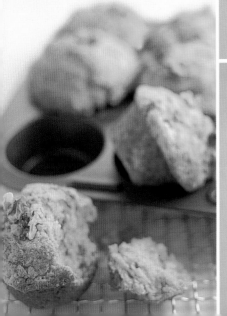

DEFICIENCY A deficiency can result from chronic alcoholism and malnutrition. Symptoms mainly include depression, headaches, confusion, numbness and tingling in the hands and feet, anaemia, skin lesions, decreased immunity and poor growth.

CAUTION Regularly taking high doses of vitamin B6 (100 mg or more per day) should be avoided because it may cause nerve damage. Make sure you check the label of B6 supplements because some contain high doses.

VITAMIN B12 (COBALAMIN)

Seafood and fish, especially clams, oysters, sardines and mussels, are a good way to get vitamin B12 and other vital nutrients.

RECOMMENDED DAILY INTAKE
Adults 2 mcg Pregnant women 3 mcg
Lactating 2.5 mcg

FOOD SOURCES	mcg per 100 grams
CLAMS, COOKED	99
LAMB'S LIVER	77
BEEF KIDNEY	51
CALVES' LIVER	36
MUSSELS, COOKED	24
CAVIAR	20
CHICKEN LIVER	19
PIG'S LIVER	19
OYSTERS, RAW	16
BEEF HEART	14
TUNA, FRESH, COOKED	11
LAMB BRAINS	9.3
SARDINES, CANNED	9
CRAB	7.3
RABBIT, LEAN, COOKED	6.5
RAINBOW TROUT	5
SALMON, FRESH	4.4
SNAPPER	3.5
SMOKED SALMON	3.3
EGG YOLK	3.1
LAMB, LEAN, COOKED	3
SKIM MILK POWDER	3
BEEF, LEAN	2.6
FLOUNDER	2.5
SWORDFISH	2
FETA CHEESE	1.7
SWISS CHEESE	1.6
BRIE CHEESE	1.6
EDAM CHEESE	1.5
HADDOCK	1.4
SQUID	1.2

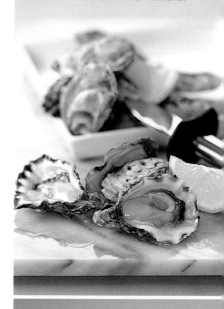

RECIPE Steam clams in a little white wine, chopped tomato, onion and garlic. Discard any that do not open. Sprinkle with a little crumbled feta and chopped fresh parsley.

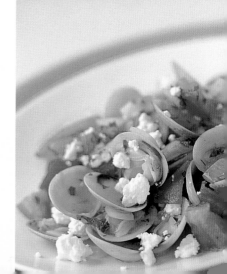

Dairy foods, especially cheeses that are ripened with bacteria, moulds or penicillin, are a good source of vitamin B12. Vegetarians can benefit from including these cheeses in their diet.

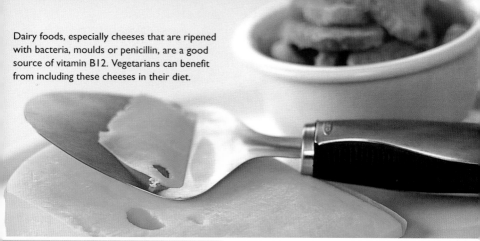

Vitamin B12 is widely available in animal foods (beef, lamb, chicken), especially liver and other organ meats, which are particularly rich sources of many vitamins.

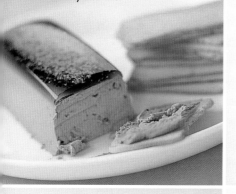

VITAMIN B12 (COBALAMIN) is

a water-soluble vitamin that is essential for growth and the production of energy from fatty acids. It is necessary for DNA synthesis and normal nerve functioning. It can be made by bacteria, fungi and algae, but not by plants and animals.

Fresh egg yolks are a good source of this vitamin, so make an eggflip for a snack.

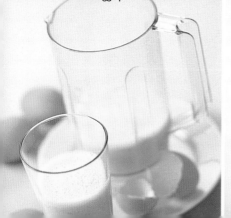

DEFICIENCY Because plant foods do not contain vitamin B12, strict vegetarians (vegans) may require B12 supplements in order to meet their requirements. They should also have regular medical checkups as it may take years for deficiency symptoms to appear.

VITAMINS – WATER-SOLUBLE
FOLATE or FOLIC ACID

REFERENCE NUTRIENT INTAKE

Women and men: 200 mcg/day.
(Pregnancy: 300 mcg/day, see also 'Extra needs' opposite. Lactation: 260 mcg/day.)

FOOD SOURCES	mcg per 100 g
Dried yeast	4000
Liver, chicken, fried	1350
Yeast extract	1150
Meat extract	1050
Soya flour	345
Wheat germ	331
Fortified breakfast cereals	150–330
Liver, lamb, fried	260
Black-eye beans, boiled	210
Sweetcorn, baby, fresh or frozen, boiled	152
Pinto beans, boiled	145
Broccoli, purple sprouting, boiled	140
Muesli, Swiss-style	140
Egg yolk	130
Brussels sprouts, boiled	110
Peanuts	110
Cheese, Camembert	102
Swiss chard, boiled	100
Pâté, liver	99
Sesame seeds	97
Spinach, boiled	90
Cheese, Stilton	77
Hazelnuts	72
Cashew nuts	67
Walnuts	66
Spring greens, boiled	66
Wholemeal rolls	62
Oatmeal	60
Green beans, boiled	57
Lettuce	55
Soya beans, boiled	54
Oranges	31

RECIPE Make the greenest of green salads with cos lettuce, lightly steamed broccoli florets, asparagus, baby spinach, soya beans and avocado. Dress with an orange, soya and walnut oil dressing to accompany a big bowl of chilli con carne.

A diet high in beans and pulses will ensure that you have high levels of folic acid. Bean salads are easy to prepare and last for up to a week in the refrigerator in an airtight container. Delicious served hot or cold.

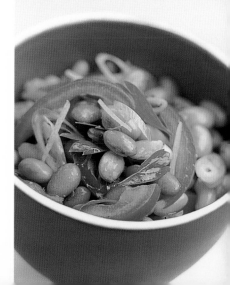

DRIED YEAST is a very rich source of folate. Adding a teaspoonful to a banana and date milkshake with a tablespoon of wheat germ is an easy way to have it.

Green leafy vegetables such as spinach, broccoli and lettuce are an excellent way to obtain folate. However, things such as cooking at high temperatures, light, and lengthy storage at room temperature will destroy it, so remember that eating the vegetables fresh and lightly steamed or stir-fried is best.

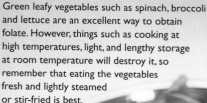

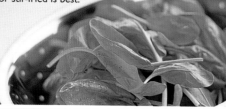

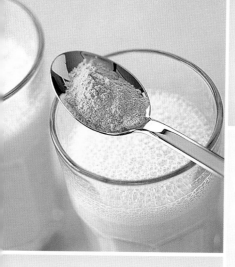

FOLATE or FOLIC ACID is a

vitamin essential for the nervous system and proper functioning of the brain. It is also necessary for growth and reproduction of body cells. It is vital for the healthy development of babies in utero. Folic acid takes its name from the Latin word for foliage or leaf.

RECIPE For a delicious folate-filled vegetable accompaniment, lightly steam purple sprouting broccoli and green beans and top with chopped hazelnuts and sunflower and sesame seeds. Drizzle with lemon-infused butter.

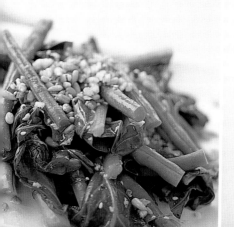

EXTRA NEEDS Though relatively rare, a severe folic acid deficiency can cause a form of anaemia (megaloblastic anaemia), a sore, red tongue, chronic diarrhoea and poor growth (in children). Low levels of folic acid intake have no symptoms but may raise the risk of heart disease and birth defects.

CAUTION Pregnant women are advised to take a 400 mcg folic acid supplement every day until the twelfth week of pregnancy. Getting sufficient folic acid is thought to reduce the risk of the baby being born with neural tube defects.

VITAMINS – WATER-SOLUBLE
VITAMIN C (ASCORBIC ACID)

REFERENCE NUTRIENT INTAKE
Women and men: 40 mg/day.
(Pregnancy: 50 mg/day. Lactation: 70 mg/day.)

RECIPE Char-grill tuna or chicken pieces and top with a salsa made with mango, tomato, red onion, chilli, and red and green peppers. Serve on finely shredded Chinese cabbage, which has been tossed with a little sesame oil, lime juice and fresh parsley.

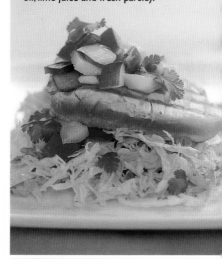

FOOD SOURCES	mg per 100 g
Guava	230
Red chillies	225
Blackcurrants	200
Parsley	190
Red peppers (capsicum)	140
Green peppers (capsicum)	120
Spring greens	77
Strawberries	77
Curly kale, boiled	71
Watercress	62
Cabbage, Savoy	62
Brussels sprouts, boiled	60
Papaya (pawpaw)	60
Kiwi	59
Red cabbage, raw	55
Oranges	54
Orange juice, freshly squeezed	48
Broccoli, boiled	44
Tomatoes, grilled	44
Cauliflower	43
Redcurrants	40
Sweetcorn, baby, fresh or frozen, boiled	39
Orange juice, unsweetened	39
Lime juice	38
Nectarines	37
Mango	37
Grapefruit	36

(continued)

RECIPE A delicious drink made with mixed berries, orange juice, papaya and ice, blended until smooth, will help boost your vitamin C intake.

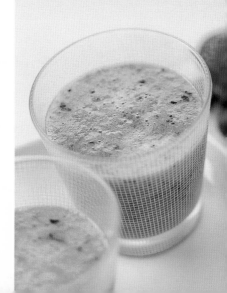

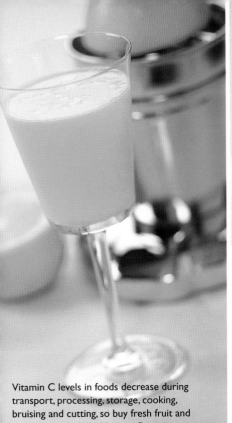

It is easy to obtain your daily vitamin C requirements by eating plenty of fruit and vegetables. The fresher they are, the more vitamins they contain, so try growing your own. Chillies and herbs grow easily.

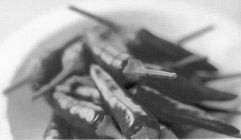

Vitamin C levels in foods decrease during transport, processing, storage, cooking, bruising and cutting, so buy fresh fruit and vegetables regularly. Vitamin C survives longer in citrus fruits than all other fruits and vegetables. Orange juice will retain its vitamin C content for up to two days if kept in an airtight container in the refrigerator.

VITAMIN C (ASCORBIC ACID) is a water-soluble vitamin

required for the formation of connective tissue such as collagen, necessary for the formation of healthy skin, bones, cartilage and teeth. Vitamin C is also needed for the synthesis of neuro-transmitters, hormones, such as thyroid and sex hormones, and carnitine needed for fatty acid breakdown.

Vitamin C is the least stable of all the vitamins and is extremely sensitive to oxygen, light, heat, and certain metals including copper and iron. Cooking reduces the vitamin C in foods by about 50 per cent. Microwaving, steaming and stir-frying help preserve vitamin C and are the most suitable cooking methods.

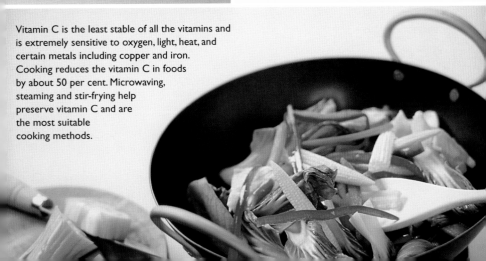

VITAMIN C (ASCORBIC ACID)

FOOD SOURCES (continued)	mg per 100 g
Salad, green	36
Raspberries	32
Red cabbage, boiled	32
Sugar snap peas	32
Grapefruit juice, unsweetened	31
Peaches	31
Tomatoes, cherry	28
Cauliflower, boiled	27
Satsumas	27
Melon, cantaloupe-type	26
Spinach	26
Spring onions	26
Gooseberries	26
Mango juice, canned	25
Liver, chicken, fried	23
Sweet potato, baked	23
Passion fruit	23
Cabbage, chinese	21
Courgette, raw	21
Coleslaw (with mayonnaise)	20
Broad beans, boiled	20
Cabbage, boiled	20
Garlic	17
Bilberries	17
Radish, red	17
Peas, boiled	16
Courgette, boiled	11

RECIPE Lightly steam broccoli, drizzle with lime juice and sesame oil and finish with oyster sauce and slices of fried garlic.

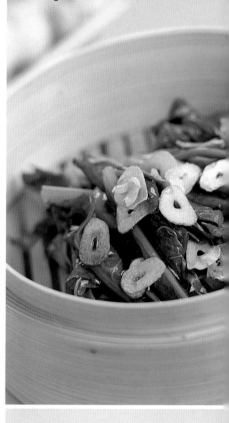

There is a limit to the amount of vitamin C our body tissues absorb at one time so it is recommended that we consume regular, small doses of it throughout the day by eating vitamin C rich foods. Any excess that the body does not use is excreted in urine.

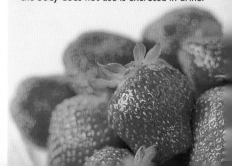

RECIPE Make a delicious sweet couscous by very gently heating 450 ml (1 pint) orange juice, then pouring it over 175 g (6 oz) of couscous. Add 1 cinnamon stick, cover and allow to stand until all the liquid is absorbed. Serve with a freshly prepared fruit salad.

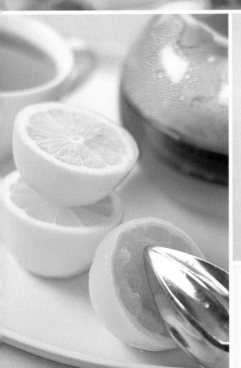

VITAMIN C (ASCORBIC ACID)

acts as an antioxidant to protect the body against damage caused by free radicals and pollutants such as cigarette smoke and air pollution. People who smoke may need to consume up to twice the RNI to maintain their vitamin C levels because their body has to use so much of it to protect the body's tissues from cigarette smoke and chemicals. Vitamin C also promotes healing and iron absorption.

DEFICIENCY Signs are increased susceptibility to infection, loss of appetite, muscle cramps, dry skin, splitting hair, bleeding gums, impaired digestion, anaemia, nosebleeds and bruising. Scurvy can occur in babies fed only cow's milk, in alcoholics and in elderly people with poor diets.

CAUTION More than 1 g a day can cause abdominal cramps, diarrhoea and nausea. More than 3 g a day can interfere with drugs that slow blood clotting, and with tests that monitor blood glucose levels. People with kidney problems or a genetic tendency to store excess iron should not take high doses.

Citrus fruits are an excellent source of vitamin C. Vitamin C stimulates the activity of the immune system and increases the breakdown of histamine, a molecule that causes inflammation. Vitamin C helps protect the body against viruses. For these reasons, it may reduce the severity of cold symptoms.

VITAMINS – WATER-SOLUBLE
BIOTIN

No RNI. Intakes between 10 and 200 mcg/day are considered adequate and safe.

FOOD SOURCES	mcg per 100 g
Liver, chicken, fried	216
Dried yeast	200
Peanuts, roasted, salted	102
Peanut butter	102
Mixed nuts	86
Almonds	64
Plaice, grilled	57
Liver, calf, fried	50
Egg yolk	50
Wheat bran	45
Liver, lamb, fried	33
Wheat germ	25
Soya beans, boiled	25
Eggs, whole	20
Oatmeal	20
Walnuts	19
Muesli, Swiss-style	15
Pâté, liver	14
Cashew nuts, plain	13
Haggis, boiled	12
Pilchards, canned in tomato sauce	11
Brazil nuts	11
Kippers, baked	10
Salmon, pink, canned in brine	9
Salmon, grilled	9
Cheese, Camembert	8
Cheese, hard	3
Milk, semi-skimmed	2
Yoghurt, whole milk, fruit	2

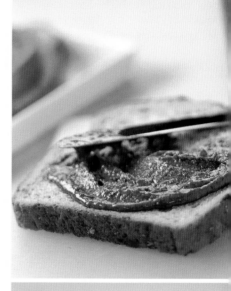

A nut spread instead of butter or margarine on bread will not only add flavour but also increase the biotin and vitamin content of your diet.

Unlike a lot of other vitamins, biotin is stable to light, heat and acid. Raw egg white contains avidin (a protein that prevents biotin absorption), but avidin is destroyed by cooking egg white.

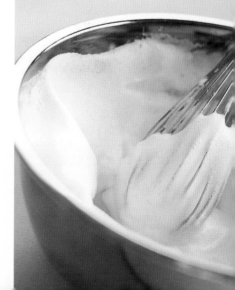

RECIPE Lightly fry thinly sliced lamb's liver in a little oil and butter with chopped onion and pieces of bacon. Thicken with some flour and a little stock, then simmer until you have a rich gravy.

Dried soya beans are available in supermarkets or health food shops. They are easy to cook. Boil them in lightly salted water and serve as a green vegetable. Canned soya beans are also available.

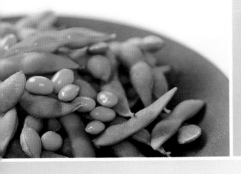

BIOTIN, a member of the B complex group, is required for cell growth and the metabolism of protein, folic acid, B5 and B12. It plays a special role in helping the body to use glucose, as well as promoting healthy hair and nails. Without biotin in the diet, the ability of the body to break down fatty foods is impaired.

RECIPE Oatmeal, wheat bran and nuts all provide biotin in the diet so why not kickstart your day with a bowl of porridge topped with wheat bran, nuts and fruit.

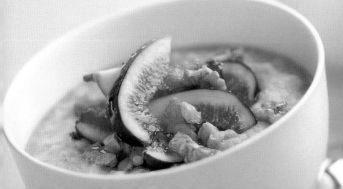

NUTRIENTS – WATER-SOLUBLE
FLAVONOIDS

No RNI. Exact values are difficult to obtain.

FOOD SOURCES

Apricots

Beetroot

Blackberries

Blackcurrants

Blueberries

Broad beans

Broccoli

Buckwheat

Cabbage

Cherries

Cranberries

Endive

Garlic

Grapefruit

Grapes

Green tea

Lemons

Limes

Mandarins

Melon

Mulberries

Onions

Oranges

Papaya (pawpaw)

Parsley

Pecans

Peppers (capsicum)

Plums

Potatoes

Prunes

Radishes

Raspberries

Rosehips

Squash

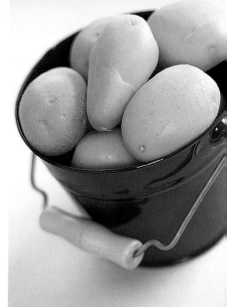

Quercetin is a flavonoid found in citrus fruits, berries, tomatoes and potatoes and may help to reduce histamine production and allergy and inflammatory symptoms.

These powerful antioxidants are found in most fruits and vegetables and this may partly explain why the regular consumption of a wide variety of fresh fruits and vegetables appears to reduce the risk of heart disease and some cancers.

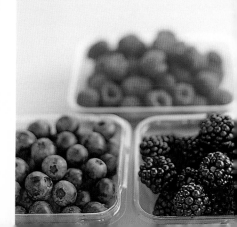

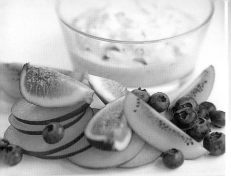

RECIPE For a flavonoid boost, serve a home-made berry yoghurt with fresh fruits, including more berries.

Flavonoids are present in many fruits so eat plenty of whole fruits and enjoy lots of freshly squeezed juice.

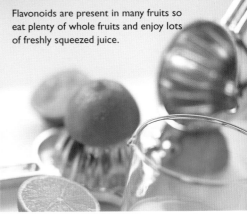

To assist your intake of flavonoids, you can substitute your afternoon cuppa with soothing green tea or replace that beer with a glass of red wine.

FLAVONOIDS are a group of phytochemicals found in all plants. More than 4000 flavonoids have been identified so far. They are antioxidants that can be found in most fruits and vegetables. They are usually found in flowers, and accompany vitamin C in the leaves and stems of brightly coloured fruits, vegetables and plants. They prevent oxidation in the tissues and mop up free radicals. They seem to be more powerful antioxidants than vitamins C, E and selenium.

RECIPE Purée cooked, peeled beetroot, add some garlic and broad beans and mix with a little stock.

FLAVONOIDS are also pigment compounds that give the red and blue colours to blueberries, raspberries and red cabbage, and the pale yellow colour in potatoes, onions and citrus rind. They are richest in the pith and peel of citrus fruit rather than juice, so add these to salads, or juice, in small quantities as they can be quite bitter.

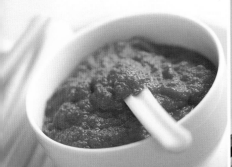

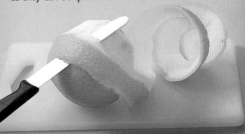

NUTRIENTS – WATER SOLUBLE
INOSITOL

No RNI. Exact values are difficult to obtain, and it can be made in the body.

FOOD SOURCES

Barley
Black-eye peas
Bread, wholemeal
Cabbage
Chickpeas
Dried yeast
Grapefruit
Lentils
Lettuce
Lima beans
Melon, cantaloupe-type
Oatmeal
Onions
Oranges
Peanut butter
Peanuts, roasted
Peas, green
Pecans
Raisins
Rice bran
Rice, brown
Rice germ
Soya flour
Soya beans
Strawberries
Watermelon
Wheat germ

Lightly cook lentils in a stock with a bay leaf and clove-studded onion. Season with salt and pepper and chopped fresh herbs. These lentils make a perfect accompaniment to any meal.

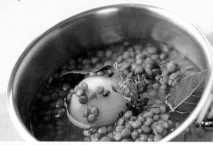

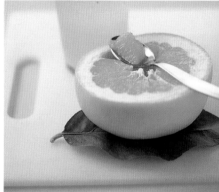

All citrus fruits except lemons, juiced or eaten in their natural form, provide inositol in generous quantities.

Lettuce and other foods on the list are all good sources of inositol as well as other vitamins and minerals.

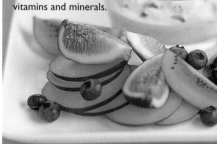

RECIPE Home-made muesli is a good way to combine foods that contain inositol. Mix oatmeal, wheat germ, rice bran, raisins and nuts. Store in an airtight container.

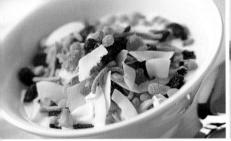

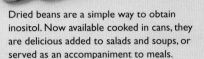

Dried beans are a simple way to obtain inositol. Now available cooked in cans, they are delicious added to salads and soups, or served as an accompaniment to meals.

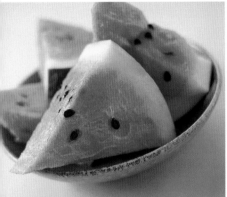

Half a cantaloupe melon, a punnet of strawberries, or a big wedge of watermelon will boost inositol levels.

Barley makes a delicious accompaniment to any meal and is as easy to cook as rice. To give it extra flavour, substitute the water with stock or the reserved liquid from rehydrated dried mushrooms.

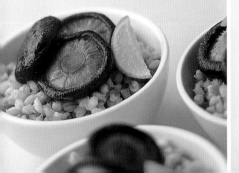

INOSITOL

INOSITOL works in a similar way to choline (see page 160) and, like choline, is not a vitamin because it can be made in the body from glucose. It is a component of the fatty compounds in cell membranes where it plays a role in relaying the messages from hormones and neuro-transmitters to the inside of the cell. It appears to be involved in the metabolism of cholesterol and fat. Inositol combines with choline to make lecithin.

DEFICIENCY Deficiency is rare and unlikely in healthy people. Inositol can be synthesised from glucose and has not been shown to be essential in the diet as it can be made in the body.

NUTRIENTS – WATER-SOLUBLE
CHOLINE

No RNI because it can be made in the body to some extent.

FOOD SOURCES

Barley
Beef
Black-eye peas
Black treacle
Brains
Cabbage
Cauliflower
Chickpeas
Dried yeast
Eggs
Egg yolk
Grape juice
Ham
Kidneys, all types
Lentils
Lettuce
Liver, all types
Oatmeal
Peanuts, roasted
Peanut butter
Pork
Potatoes
Rice, brown
Soya beans
Spinach
Split peas
Sweet potatoes
Textured Vegetable Protein (TVP)
Veal
Wheat bran
Wheat germ

Lecithin is the richest source of choline and is used as a food additive in ice cream, margarine, chocolate, mayonnaise and baked goods to keep the oil separating from the other ingredients (as an emulsifying agent).

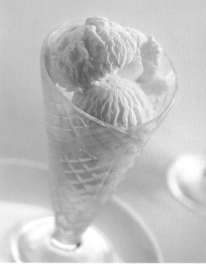

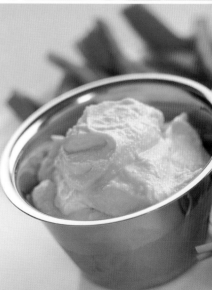

A bowl of houmous served with steamed green vegetable crudités is a great nutritious snack when studying – choline is responsible for a chemical in the brain that aids memory.

RECIPE Whisk together eggs, milk and grated Cheddar. Season with salt and pepper, add finely shredded spinach leaves and chunks of steamed sweet potato. Bake until set.

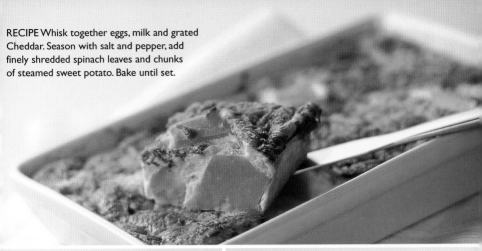

One egg will provide you with roughly enough choline for one day.

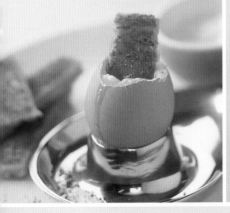

CHOLINE is not classified as a vitamin because it can be made in the body to some extent, but there is evidence that it is essential in the diet during certain stages of life. It is required for the synthesis of the neurotransmitter, acetylcholine, which is involved in nerve and brain functioning and memory. Deficiency is rare but causes liver problems.

A ham and egg sandwich using wholemeal bread will help add some of this essential compound to your diet.

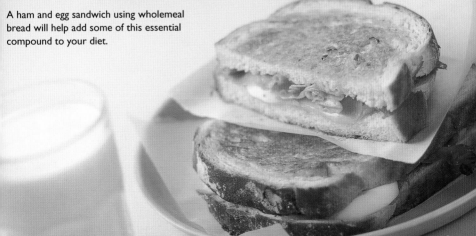

MINERALS

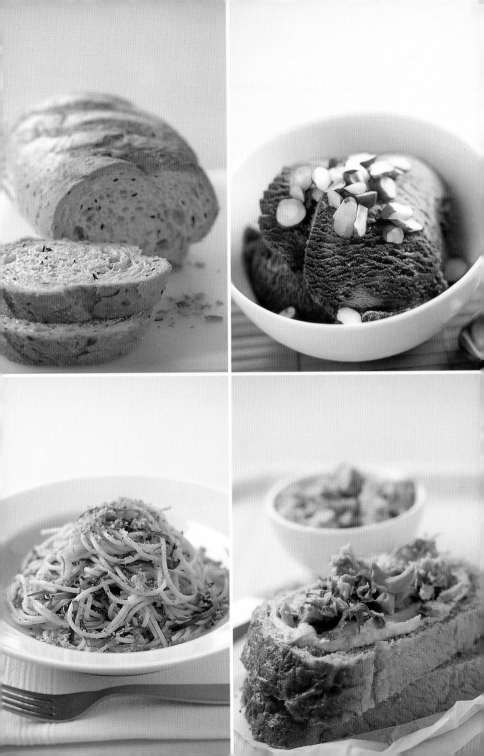

MINERALS – MAJOR
CALCIUM

REFERENCE NUTRIENT INTAKE
Women and men: 700 mg/day.
(Lactation: 1250 mg/day.)

FOOD SOURCES	mg per 100 g
Cheese, Parmesan	1200
Cheese, Emmental	970
Cheese, Gruyère	950
Cheese, Edam	770
Cheese, Cheddar	720
Tahini	680
Sesame seeds	670
Pesto sauce	560
Cheese, Brie	540
Sardines, canned in brine	540
Tofu, soya bean, steamed	510
Malted milk powder	430
Seaweed, nori, dried	430
Salmon, pink, canned, flesh and bone	300
Carob powder	390
Evaporated milk, whole	290
Almonds	240
Figs, ready-to-eat	230
Chocolate, milk	220
Soya flour	210
Parsley	200
Yoghurt, low fat, plain	190
Spinach	170
Watercress	170
Curly kale, boiled	150
Tortilla chips	150
Greek yoghurt	150
Muffins	140
Hazelnuts	140
Oysters	140
Vanilla ice cream	130

(continued)

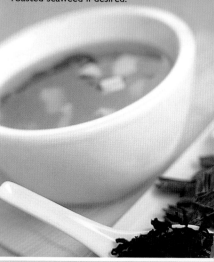

RECIPE Kelp, wakame and nori are varieties of seaweed used in Japanese cooking. To make a quick miso soup, simmer kelp, miso and dashi granules for 10 minutes before adding small cubes of tofu. Sprinkle with strips of roasted seaweed if desired.

Calcium is most readily absorbed from dairy products because lactose (milk sugar) enhances calcium absorption. If you are lactose intolerant, you may still be able to tolerate 2–3 servings of dairy, consumed in small quantities over a day. Full-cream milk may be easier to digest than skimmed.

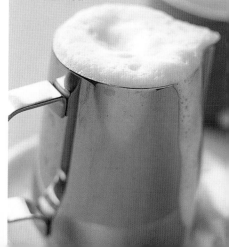

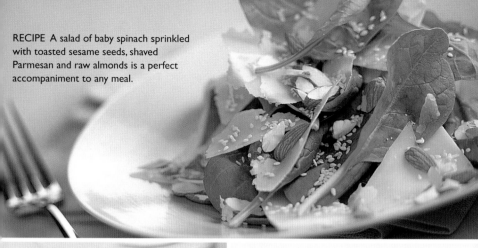

RECIPE A salad of baby spinach sprinkled with toasted sesame seeds, shaved Parmesan and raw almonds is a perfect accompaniment to any meal.

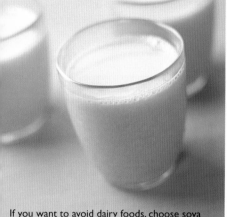

If you want to avoid dairy foods, choose soya milk products fortified with calcium.

CALCIUM is the most abundant mineral in the body and works with phosphorus and other elements to give strength to bones and teeth. Calcium is necessary for blood clotting and the transmission of nerve impulses. It is essential in enzyme regulation, in the secretion of insulin in adults, and in the regulation of muscle function. Vitamin D is required for calcium absorption.

Contrary to popular belief, there is no need for extra calcium during pregnancy. This is because a woman's body becomes more efficient at absorbing calcium during pregnancy. More is recommended during breast-feeding as a precaution. Children and adolescents need to make sure they are getting enough calcium to ensure growth. Cheese is one of the richest sources of calcium. Try Swiss cheeses, such as Emmental.

CALCIUM

FOOD SOURCES (continued)	mg per 100 g
Tempeh	120
Pineapple, dried	120
Wheat germ bread	120
Milk, skimmed or semi-skimmed	120
Milk, whole	115
White bread	110
Broccoli, purple sprouting	110
Prawns, boiled	110
Currant buns	110
Sunflower seeds	110
Cream crackers	110
Scones, wholemeal	110
Cottage cheese, plain	110
Muesli Swiss-style	110
Cream cheese	98
Walnuts	94
Cream, fresh, soured	93
Apricots, dried	92
Fish fingers, cod, grilled	92
Cream, fresh, single	91
Fromage frais, plain	89
Tzatziki	88
Mackerel, canned in tomato sauce	82
Miso	73
Red kidney beans, canned	71
Haricot beans, boiled	65
Sultanas	64
Pecan nuts	61
Eggs, whole, raw or poached	57
Broccoli	56
Oatmeal	55
Sugar snap peas	54
Baked beans, canned in tomato sauce	53
Oranges	47
Chickpeas, boiled	46

Fresh or canned sardines, if eaten with the bones, are a rich source of calcium. Drizzle with lemon juice and sprinkle with plenty of cracked black pepper.

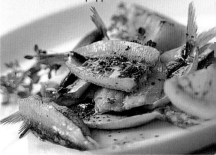

Calcium is required for blood clotting, muscle contraction and nerve function. Although the calcium in spinach and other vegetables isn't as well absorbed as the calcium in dairy foods, it can still provide you with some calcium as well as other vital nutrients.

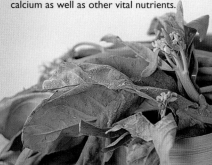

Calcium absorption is enhanced by lactose, the natural sugar present in milk and dairy products, so calcium in dairy products is easily absorbed. A big bowl of yoghurt is an easy calcium-rich snack.

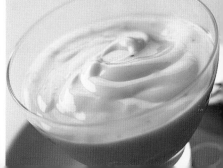

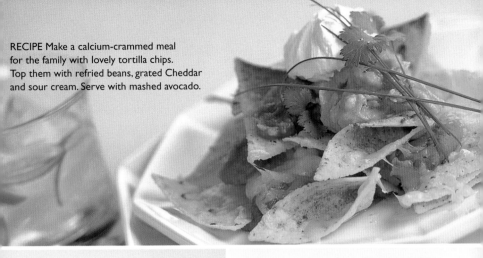

RECIPE Make a calcium-crammed meal for the family with lovely tortilla chips. Top them with refried beans, grated Cheddar and sour cream. Serve with mashed avocado.

Nuts and seeds are a good source of calcium, especially sesame seeds which can be used to coat foods, add flavour to salads, or used as tahini paste as a spread for bread.

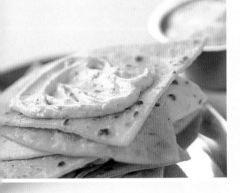

Next time you are baking, try substituting carob powder for cocoa powder to add more calcium to the product.

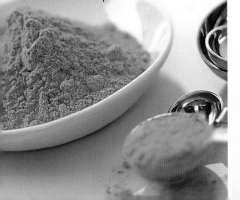

CALCIUM As children, teenagers and young adults, bones not only grow in length and width, they also become more dense as the amount of calcium and other minerals they contain increase. This makes them strong and the stronger they are, the less likely they are to fracture and break. Provided we get enough calcium, bone density will increase until our late 20s or early 30s, when it will reach its peak. From then on, more bone cells are removed than are replaced and because of this, bone gets thinner as we get older. This is a normal part of ageing, but if you have a low peak bone mass, you may lose more bone cells as you age and develop osteoporosis (brittle bone disease) in later life. Oestrogen helps to maintain calcium in the bones, so bone loss is accelerated in women after the menopause. Even though peak bone mass is reached in early life, it is important to maintain an adequate calcium intake as you get older.

DEFICIENCY Signs of calcium deficiency include osteoporosis, osteomalacia, muscle spasms and cramping, heart palpitations, high blood pressure, rickets and joint pain. Most people would not benefit from calcium supplements as it is not difficult to get enough from diet alone.

MINERALS – MAJOR
MAGNESIUM

Magnesium is found in green leafy vegetables, so add some wilted spinach to pasta dishes, salads and sandwiches.

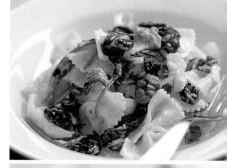

REFERENCE NUTRIENT INTAKE
Women: 270 mg/day.
(Lactation: 320 mg/day.)
Men: 300 mg/day.

FOOD SOURCES	mg per 100 g
Wheat bran	520
Cocoa powder	520
Seaweed, dried, wakame	470
Brazil nuts	410
Sunflower seeds	390
Tahini	380
Sesame seeds	310
Winkles, boiled	340
Wheat germ	270
Cashew nuts, plain	270
Almonds	270
Pine nuts	270
Dried yeast	230
Peanuts	210
Peanut butter	180
Oat and wheat bran	180
Black treacle	180
Walnuts	160
Yeast extract	160
Hazelnuts	160
Shrimps, boiled	110
Crispbread, rye	100
Mustard, wholegrain	93
Swiss chard, boiled	86
Figs, dried	80
Wholemeal bread	76
Tempeh	70
Apricots, dried	65
Soya beans, boiled	63
Houmous	62
Prawns, boiled	49
Spinach, boiled	34
Tofu	23

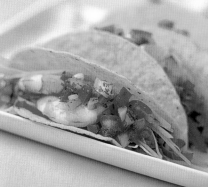

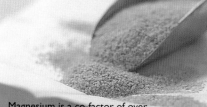

RECIPE Prawn or tofu tacos filled with shredded spinach, tomato, carrot and salsa.

Magnesium is a co-factor of over 300 enzymes needed for vital processes such as the production of energy from carbohydrates, fat and protein, and DNA synthesis. An easy way to add magnesium to your diet is to snack on dried fruit or nut mixes or sprinkle generous tablespoons of wheat germ on breakfast cereal or yoghurt.

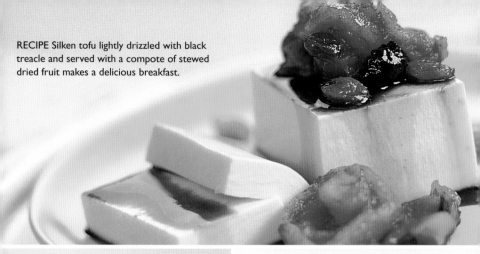

RECIPE Silken tofu lightly drizzled with black treacle and served with a compote of stewed dried fruit makes a delicious breakfast.

Magnesium is involved in regulating calcium balance in the body and is needed for the action of vitamin D and many hormones, so eat plenty of foods containing magnesium.

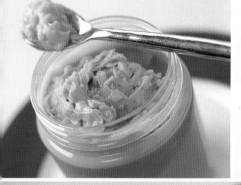

MAGNESIUM, along with calcium and phosphorus, is needed for strong, healthy bones and proper nerve and muscle functioning. It is essential for the action of vitamin D, and hence, calcium absorption, and many hormones. Symptoms of low levels of magnesium in the body are muscle spasms, tremors, cramping, twitching, changes in blood pressure and heartbeat. It is difficult to get too much magnesium as the absorption decreases as intake increases and the kidneys are very efficient at eliminating any excess.

RECIPE Sesame and sunflower seeds are a rich source of magnesium. Combined with crushed almonds, pine nuts and cashews and mixed with ricotta and herbs, they make a delicious filling for veal, chicken or pork, or can be sprinkled on baked mushrooms.

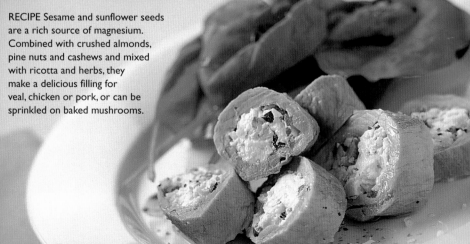

MINERALS – MAJOR
PHOSPHORUS

REFERENCE NUTRIENT INTAKE
Women and men: 550 mg/day.
(Lactation: 990 mg/day.)

FOOD SOURCES	mg per 100 g
Dried yeast	1290
Wheat bran	1200
Wheat germ	1050
Processed cheese, smoked	1030
Yeast extract	950
Pumpkin seeds	850
Cheese spread	790
Sesame seeds	720
Pine nuts	650
Sunflower seeds	640
Cheese, Gruyère	610
Brazil nuts	590
Cheese, Emmental	590
Cashew nuts	560
Almonds	550
Sardines, canned in oil	520
Egg yolk	500
Cheese, Cheddar	490
Pesto sauce	480
Monkfish, grilled	480
Pâté, liver	450
Kipper, baked	430
Kidney, pig, fried	430
Sardines, canned in tomato sauce	420
Liver, calf, fried	380
Walnuts	380
Oatmeal	380
Peanut butter	370
Kidney, lamb, fried	350
Chicken breast, grilled, no skin	310
Cheese, Feta	280
Milk	92

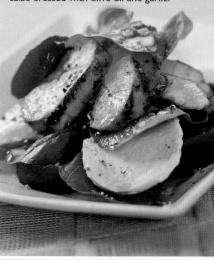

RECIPE Char-grill chicken breast fillets that have been marinated in lemon juice or vinegar, sesame seeds, garlic and kecap manis. Cook until tender, then serve sliced on a rocket, goat's cheese and beetroot salad dressed with olive oil and garlic.

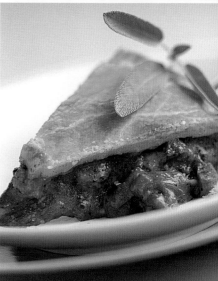

Protein-rich foods are high in phosphorus, with offal containing greater levels than a steak. Steak and kidney pie is a delicious way of sneaking offal into your diet.

RECIPE For a phosphorus-rich vegetarian meal, pan-fry or barbecue mushrooms, top with chunks of marinated feta with a little of its oil and finish with canned spicy Mexican beans.

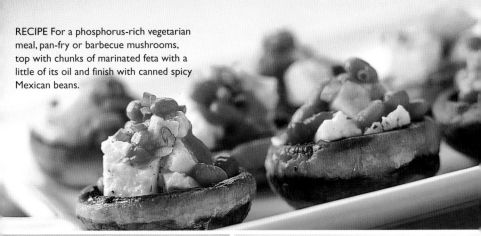

RECIPE Roast unsalted pumpkin seeds in a little honey and black sesame seeds for 15 minutes in a moderate oven. This simple snack is a good way to obtain phosphorus.

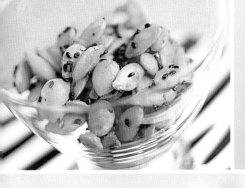

PHOSPHORUS is the second most abundant mineral in the body after calcium. It is present in every cell of the body and has important structural roles. Teamed with calcium, it is necessary for bone strength. Phosphorus is required for almost every chemical reaction in the body and for energy production. Deficiency is rare because it's in a variety of foods – even more than calcium.

Phosphorus is easily absorbed by the body; more easily even than calcium. Some dairy products, including low-fat varieties, contain relatively large amounts of phosphorus.

MINERALS – MAJOR
SODIUM

REFERENCE NUTRIENT INTAKE
Women and men: 1600 mg/day

FOOD SOURCES	mg per 100 g
Salt	39300
Bicarbonate of soda	38700
Stock cubes	10300
Soy sauce	7120
Instant gravy granules	6330
Meat extract	4370
Yeast extract	4300
Shrimps, boiled	3840
Miso	3650
Instant soup powder	3440
Bacon, back, grilled	2240
Olives in brine	2000
Ham, gammon, grilled	1930
Salmon, smoked	1880
Salami	1800
Tomato ketchup	1630
Prawns, boiled	1590
Cheese, feta	1440
Butter	750
Houmous	670
Cheese, Cheddar	670
Digestive biscuits	660
Wholemeal bread	550
White bread	520
Sardines, canned in oil	450
Cottage cheese	380
Lobster, boiled	330
Scallops, steamed	180
Eggs, boiled	140
Yoghurt, low-fat, plain	83
Milk, skimmed and whole	55

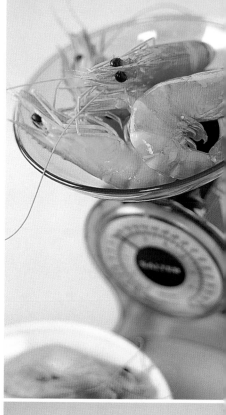

Seafood is a natural source of sodium. Shellfish contain higher levels than fish, and fresh is best as a lot of canned seafood has sodium chloride added during processing.

Most people, especially those suffering from high blood pressure, need to limit the amount of sodium in their diet. To achieve this, eliminate the use of table salt, buy salt-reduced products and keep a close eye on the amount of processed foods you eat.

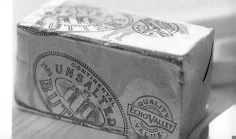

RECIPE Remove scallops from their shells and pan-fry in a little olive oil. Place some shredded fresh spinach on the cleaned shells, top with a scallop and serve with crumbled feta cheese and finely diced char-grilled marinated peppers.

Excessive perspiration, prolonged diarrhoea and vomiting increase the body's need for sodium. Electrolyte sports drinks are a simple way of gaining sodium. Contrary to popular belief, taking salt tablets will not stop cramps, so if you are healthy, don't take them. It is a lack of fluid that causes stitches and cramps.

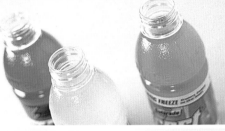

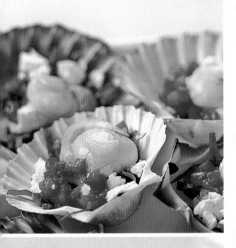

SODIUM works with potassium and chloride to regulate the acid and fluid balance in the body. It is necessary for proper muscle and nerve functioning and for maintaining a normal heartbeat. Table salt contains about 40 per cent sodium and 60 per cent chloride and its chemical name is sodium chloride. Most people in western countries eat more salt than they need and deficiency is rare.

CAUTION Currently we eat an average of 12 g salt every day. Our bodies need much less than this (about 4 g). Eating too much salt increases the amount of fluid that you retain in your body. This raises blood pressure – a major risk factor for heart disease and strokes. About three-quarters of our salt intake comes from processed foods, such as cured or smoked meats, meat products, bottled sauces and condiments, canned soups, processed cheese, crisps and salty snacks. Food labels do not usually give salt content, but the chemical name for salt is sodium chloride, and values for sodium are usually given on nutrition labels. 1 g of sodium is equivalent to about 1.5 g salt.

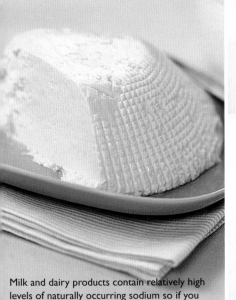

Milk and dairy products contain relatively high levels of naturally occurring sodium so if you consume dairy products you really don't need to add salt to your meals.

MINERALS – MAJOR
POTASSIUM

REFERENCE NUTRIENT INTAKE
Women and men: 3500 mg/day.

FOOD SOURCES	mg per 100 g
Yeast extract	2100
Dried yeast	2000
Apricots, dried	1880
Treacle, black	1760
Wheat bran	1160
Peaches, dried	1100
Sultanas	1060
Raisins	1020
Wheat germ	950
Pine nuts	780
Almonds	780
Parsley	760
Hazelnuts	730
Sunflower seeds	710
Dates, dried	700
Peanuts	760
Brazil nuts	660
Potatoes, baked with skin	630
Garlic	620
Coriander	540
Red snapper, fried	460
Avocados	450
Walnuts	450
Trout, rainbow, grilled	410
Bananas	400
Tempeh	370
Tuna, canned in oil	260
Yoghurt, plain	250
Carrots	170
Oranges	150
Milk, whole	140
Spinach, boiled	120
Apples	120

A cup of dried fruits is a simple way of getting your daily supply of potassium. Eaten as they are, or lightly simmered in apple juice, with spices, they make a tasty low-fat dessert or breakfast treat.

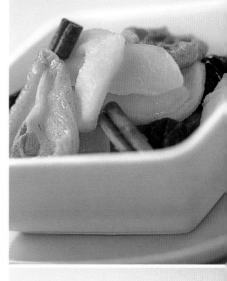

RECIPE Vegetarians can obtain generous amounts of potassium by including tempeh in their diets. It can be marinated in low-salt soy, garlic, ginger and then steamed, fried or barbecued and served on steamed greens.

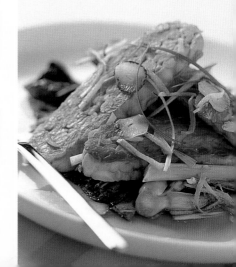

If you are prone to high blood pressure, decrease your sodium intake while increasing your potassium intake by eating more fruits and vegetables. Aim for at least five portions of fruit and vegetables every day.

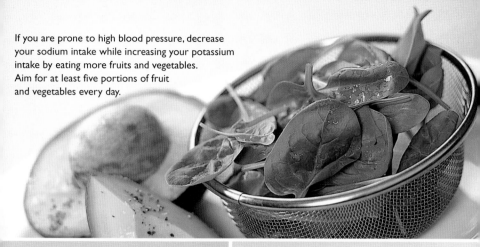

Bananas contain plenty of potassium so make them a part of your daily diet.

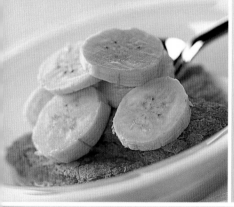

POTASSIUM, just like sodium, is necessary for maintaining the body's fluid balance, proper muscle and nerve function, and the metabolism of protein and carbohydrates. Potassium is present in many foods, so deficiency is unlikely. Potassium salt should not be used instead of table salt as a way of reducing sodium intake as it is very dangerous, especially for children.

RECIPE Seafood, especially snapper, is a rich source of potassium. Bake a whole snapper, then top it with a rich sauce of chopped herbs, pine nuts and garlic mixed with butter that has been combined with shredded lemon rind.

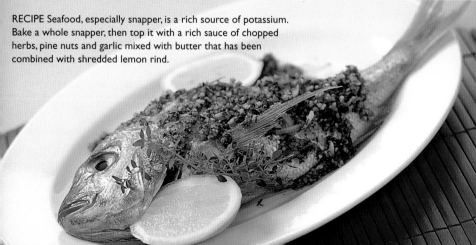

MINERALS – MAJOR
CHLORIDE

REFERENCE NUTRIENT INTAKE
Women and men: 2500 mg/day.

FOOD SOURCES	mg per 100 g
Salt	59900
Stock cubes	16000
Soy sauce	10640
Yeast extract	6630
Olives in brine	3750
Bacon back, grilled	2780
Prawns, boiled	2550
Cheese, Danish blue	1950
Cheese, Parmesan	1820
Cheese, Edam	1570
Cheese, Camembert	1120
Cheese, Cheddar	1030
Bread, white	820
Oysters	820
Sardines, canned in brine	810
Salmon, canned in brine	730
Peanuts, roasted and salted	660
Peanut butter	540
Tuna, canned in oil	530

Chlorine is often added to water for purification purposes as it prevents the growth of waterborne diseases, such as typhoid and hepatitis. Boiling the water evaporates the chlorine and may improve the taste.

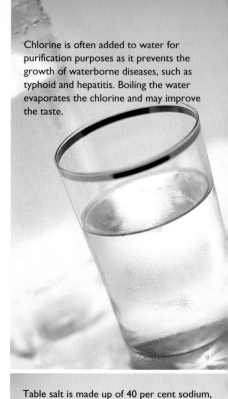

Table salt is made up of 40 per cent sodium, 60 per cent chloride. Most people get more than enough chloride from salt that is naturally present in foods and that which is added to processed foods as a preservative.

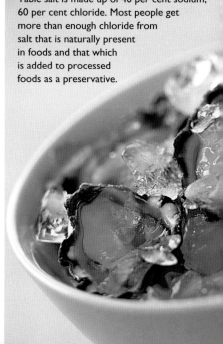

RECIPE Fill white bread with sliced Edam cheese, grilled bacon and a fried egg. Top with tomato sauce.

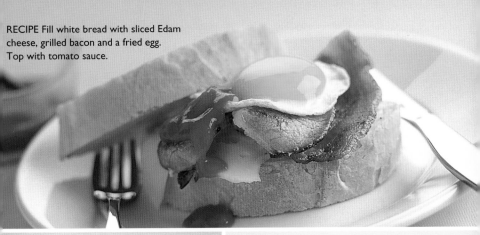

Chloride is combined with hydrogen in the stomach to make hydrochloric acid, which is essential for food digestion. Cheddar cheese is a good way to add chloride to your diet.

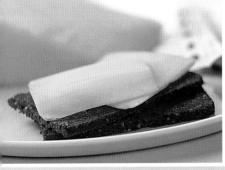

CHLORIDE, along with sodium and potassium, is important for maintaining the body's fluid balance and is therefore needed for normal muscle and nerve functioning. Virtually all of the chlorine found in foods and in our body is in the form of chloride. Deficiency is rare and only occurs when there are large losses through prolonged periods of vomiting, diarrhoea and profuse sweating.

Ripe olives stored in brine are a good way of getting chloride into your diet. Enjoy them on their own or add them to salads.

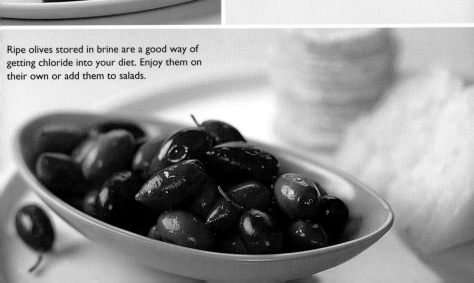

MINERALS – MAJOR
SULPHUR

No RNI. Most comes from the proteins we eat.

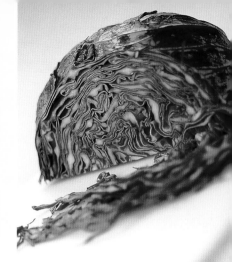

FOOD SOURCES	mcg per 100 g
Mustard powder	1280
Partridge, roast	400
Peanuts, plain	380
Cod, dried, salted, boiled	370
Peanut butter	360
Goose, roast	320
Bacon, gammon, lean, fried	310
Pork, loin, lean, grilled	310
Liver, calf, fried	300
Turkey, roast	290
Brazil nuts	290
Kidney, lamb, fried	290
Bacon, lean, grilled	290
Kipper, baked	280
Beef steak, lean, grilled	280
Mixed nuts	280
Liver, lamb, fried	270
Duck, roast	270
Chicken, lean, roast	260
Liver, chicken, fried	250
Cheese, Parmesan	250
Peaches, dried	240
Cheese, hard	230
Cheese, Stilton	230
Eggs, fried	200
Salmon, steamed	190
Egg, poached or boiled	180
Almonds	150
Walnuts	140
White bread rolls	130
Brussels sprouts	78
Red kidney beans	65
Red cabbage, boiled	54

Vegetarians who do not eat any eggs or dairy products can boost sulphur levels by eating nuts, beans and vegetables from the Brassica family, such as cabbage and Brussels sprouts.

RECIPE Cut pockets in chicken breast fillets, beat until thin with a mallet, then fill the pockets with Stilton cheese and pan-fry over medium heat until cooked through. Serve with steamed greens.

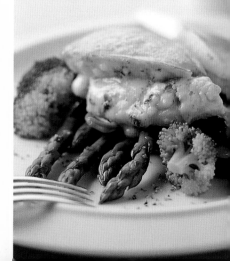

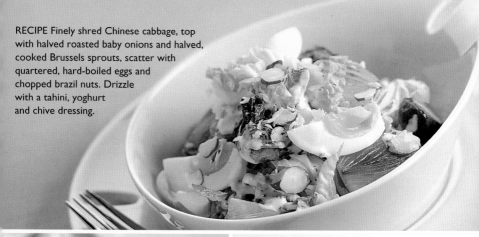

RECIPE Finely shred Chinese cabbage, top with halved roasted baby onions and halved, cooked Brussels sprouts, scatter with quartered, hard-boiled eggs and chopped brazil nuts. Drizzle with a tahini, yoghurt and chive dressing.

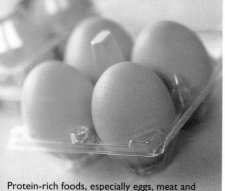

SULPHUR is known as the 'beauty mineral' as it is essential for healthy glossy skin, hair and nails. Sulphur helps regulate the acid/alkali balance in the body. Sulphur-containing amino acids are needed for protein synthesis, cell protection and detoxification.

Protein-rich foods, especially eggs, meat and fish, are high in sulphur. If you have a diet with adequate protein you'll be meeting your sulphur requirements.

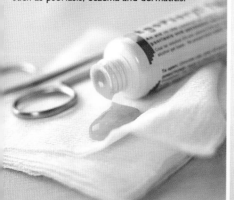

Sulphur-based creams and ointments may benefit those who suffer from skin problems such as psoriasis, eczema and dermatitis.

DEFICIENCY This is rare because we obtain most of our sulphur from proteins in the diet and it is also found in some preservatives.

CAUTION People who suffer from allergic reactions to food containing sulphur should avoid packaged dried fruit, which contains sulphur as a preservative. Look for sulphur-free varieties in health food stores.

MINERALS – TRACE
IRON

REFERENCE NUTRIENT INTAKE
Women 18 to 50 years: 14.8mg/day.
Women 50+ years: 8.7mg/day.
Men: 8.7mg/day.

FOOD SOURCES	mg per 100 g
Cockles, boiled	28
Black treacle	21.3
Fortified breakfast cereals	2–20
Seaweed, nori, dried	19.6
Wheat bran	19.2
Mussels, canned or bottled	13.0
Liver, calf, fried	12.2
Liver, chicken, fried	11.3
Kidney, lamb, fried	11.2
Liver, lamb, fried	10.9
Tahini	10.6
Cocoa powder	10.5
Sesame seeds	10.4
Winkles, boiled	10.2
Pumpkin seeds	10.4
Wheat germ	8.5
Meat extract	8.1
Clams, canned in brine	8.0
Parsley	7.7
Pâté, liver	7.4
Mussels, boiled	6.8
Peaches, dried	6.8
Sunflower seeds	6.4
Cashew nuts	6.2
Egg yolk	6.1
Lime pickle	5.8
Oysters	5.7
Pine nuts	5.6
Blackcurrants, canned in juice	5.2
Cous cous	5.0
Bulgar wheat	4.9

(continued)

Cooking for prolonged periods at high temperatures reduces the amount of iron in food, so choose cuts of meat or fish that can be steamed, poached or char-grilled, and try to get used to eating meat medium-rare.

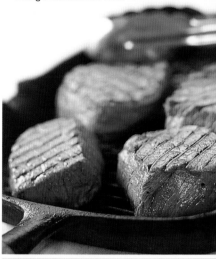

RECIPE Tofu provides some iron for vegetarians and can be enjoyed in a sweet or savoury meal. Serve silken firm tofu drizzled with a combination of sweet chilli sauce, sesame oil and soy sauce. Top with shredded, roasted nori.

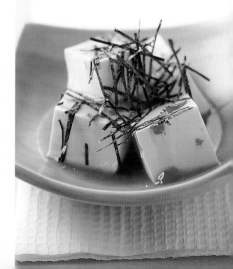

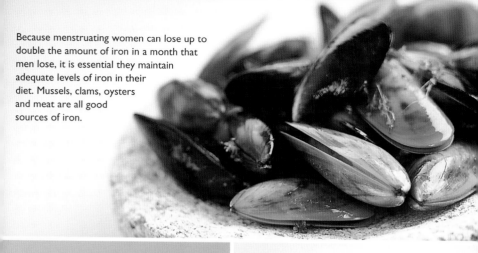

Because menstruating women can lose up to double the amount of iron in a month that men lose, it is essential they maintain adequate levels of iron in their diet. Mussels, clams, oysters and meat are all good sources of iron.

People who consume large quantities of tea or coffee need to be aware that they retard iron absorption. Substitute these with a fruit juice; it is high in vitamin C which increases absorption of iron.

IRON in the body is essential for the delivery of oxygen to cells. It is a component of the two oxygen-carrying proteins, haemoglobin and myoglobin. Most of the iron in the body is in haemoglobin in red blood cells, which transports oxygen to cells and carries carbon dioxide away. Myoglobin is in muscles, where it stores oxygen to be used during physical activity.

Offal and red meat contain a form of iron (haem iron) that is easily absorbed by the body. Current healthy eating guidelines recommend that we eat a maximum of 90 g/day of red meat and processed meats.

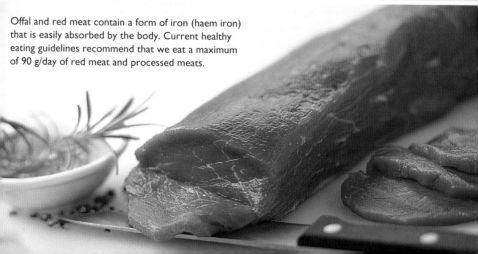

IRON

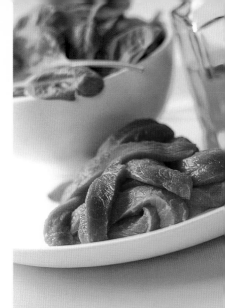

FOOD SOURCES (continued)	mg per 100 g
Miso	4.2
Apricots, dried	4.1
Raisins	3.8
Lentils, boiled	3.5
Tofu, steamed, fried	3.5
Hazelnuts	3.2
Sardines, canned in oil	3.1
Almonds	3.0
Soya beans, boiled	3.0
Walnuts	2.9
Prunes	2.9
Sardines, canned in tomato sauce	2.9
Wholemeal bread	2.7
Haricot beans, boiled	2.5
Peanut butter	2.5
Peanuts	2.5
Chocolate, plain	2.3
Swiss chard, boiled	2.3
Beef fillet, lean, grilled	2.3
Watercress	2.2
Eggs, fried	2.2
Sultanas	2.2
Spinach	2.1
Chickpeas, boiled	2.1
Curly kale, boiled	2.0
Red kidney beans, canned	2.0
Houmous	1.9
Eggs, boiled	1.9
Spinach, boiled	1.6
Peas, boiled	1.5
Pork fillet, lean, grilled	1.3
Broccoli, boiled	1.0
Tuna, canned in brine	1.0
Chicken, roast	0.7
Asparagus, boiled	0.6
Salmon, grilled	0.5
Brown rice, boiled	0.5

There are two types of iron in foods. Haem iron is in meat and meat products. Non-haem iron is in plant foods. Haem iron is much more readily absorbed than non-haem iron.

Foods containing vitamin C will increase iron absorption of non-haem iron so it is wise to include these foods with iron-rich meals. Try adding peppers to stir-fries and stews.

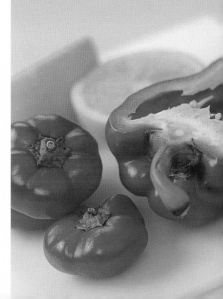

RECIPE Char-grill rump steak until medium-rare, slice and serve on a bed of baby spinach topped with sliced char-grilled red capsicum and parsley pesto.

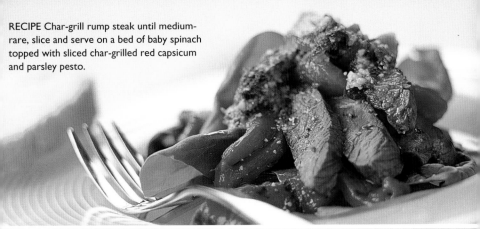

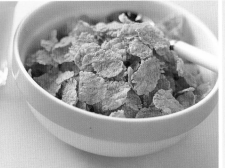

A bowl of muesli or iron-fortified breakfast cereal and a glass of orange juice each morning is a good start as the presence of vitamin C in the meal can enhance the absorption of iron.

IRON deficiency is the most common nutrient deficiency and many people have reduced iron stores. Deficiency impairs mood, ability to concentrate and physical performance, and can lead to anaemia. People who are most at risk of developing iron deficiency are women (particularly when pregnant), infants, fussy eaters, athletes and vegetarians.

Factors inhibiting iron absorption include phytates, calcium, soya protein and cooking at high temperature for prolonged periods. This doesn't mean you should avoid foods such as milk but try to have them separately from foods rich in iron.

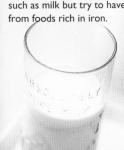

DEFICIENCY Symptoms include fatigue, poor circulation, depression, reduced recovery from exercise, reduced physical and mental performance and anaemia.

CAUTION Never take high-dose supplements unless under medical supervision. People with haemochromatosis, which makes them absorb iron very efficiently, should not increase intake.

CAUTION Children under six years can mistake red iron supplements for sweets. Accidental overdose of just five pills leads to death, so store supplements away from children.

MINERALS – TRACE
ZINC

REFERENCE NUTRIENT INTAKE
Women: 7 mg/day.
(Lactation: 9.5 to 13 mg/day.)
Men: 9.5 mg/day.

FOOD SOURCES	mg per 100 g
Oysters	59.2
Wheat germ	17.0
Wheat bran	16.2
Liver, calf, fried	15.9
Whelks, boiled	12.1
Beef braising steak, lean, braised	9.5
Yeast, dried	8.0
Quorn myco-protein	7.5
Pumpkin seeds	6.6
Pine nuts	6.5
Liver, lamb, fried	5.9
Cashew nuts	5.9
Crab, canned in brine	5.7
Beef mince, extra lean, stewed	5.8
Crab, boiled	5.5
Pecan nuts	5.3
Cheese, Parmesan	5.3
Sesame seeds	5.3
Cheese, Emmental	4.4
Brazil nuts	4.2
Curry powder	4.1
Oat and wheat bran	4.0
Egg yolk	3.9
Kidney, lamb, fried	3.6
Miso	3.3
Anchovies, canned in oil	3.5
Pork fillet, lean, grilled	2.7
Cheese, Cheddar	2.3
Chicken, breast, grilled, no skin	0.8
Tofu, steamed	0.7
Milk, whole	0.4

RECIPE Children need zinc for normal growth. Adolescents who have acne may benefit from increasing the zinc in their diet. Prepare a burger with a wholewheat roll, lettuce, home-made minced steak, Cheddar cheese and tomato slices, grated carrot and fried egg.

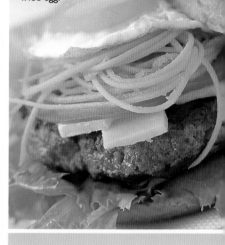

Vegetarians may struggle to find foods rich in zinc that is easily absorbed. A delicious miso udon noodle soup topped with shredded nori and cubed tofu will help with zinc intake.

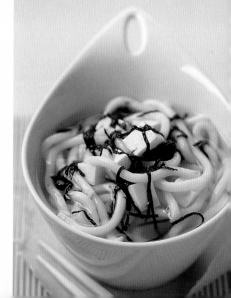

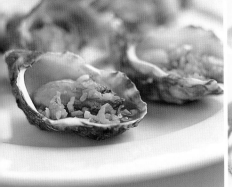

Oysters win hands down when it comes to zinc. Enjoy them natural or topped with your favourite sauce and grilled.

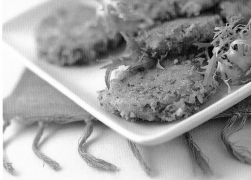

RECIPE Prepare crab cakes using canned crab, mashed potato, a pinch of curry powder, fresh herbs and grated Cheddar cheese.

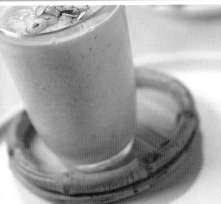

RECIPE In your blender, make a drink using skimmed milk powder, oat bran, wheat germ, hazelnuts and fresh mango.

ZINC wears many hats. It is required to assist our appetite as well as our sense of smell and taste. It helps fight infections, improves immunity, maintains healthy nails, skin, hair, tissue growth and repair, and is necessary for sexual development and reproduction. Zinc is involved in the action of many enzymes that control various chemical reactions in the body.

Beef is one of the best dietary sources of zinc. Spaghetti bolognese or a beef stir-fry are delicious ways to keep it in the diet.

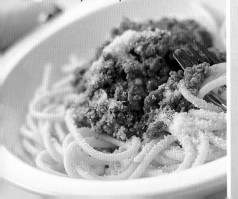

DEFICIENCY Signs are loss of taste, smell and appetite, poor growth and wound healing, reduced libido and sperm count, late onset of puberty, dry flaky skin, dandruff, and increased susceptibility to infection. People at risk of deficiency include alcoholics, vegans, children and elderly people with poor diets.

CAUTION Zinc supplements can result in toxicity problems such as gastrointestinal irritation, decreased immunity and reduced copper absorption. Supplements containing more than 50 mg of elemental zinc should be avoided as they may cause nausea, headaches and decreased copper absorption.

MINERALS – TRACE
COPPER

REFERENCE NUTRIENT INTAKE
Women and men: 1.2mg/day.
(Lactation: 1.5mg/day.)

FOOD SOURCES	mg per 100 g
Liver, calf, fried	23.9
Liver, lamb, fried	13.5
Oysters	7.5
Whelks, boiled	6.6
Dried yeast	5.0
Cocoa powder	3.9
Tomato puree	2.9
Sunflower seeds	2.3
Cashew nuts	2.1
Shrimps, boiled	1.9
Crab, boiled	1.8
Brazil nuts	1.8
Winkles, boiled	1.7
Pumpkin seeds	1.6
Sesame seeds	1.5
Tahini	1.5
Lobster, boiled	1.4
Walnuts	1.3
Pine nuts	1.3
Hazelnuts	1.2
Pecan nuts	1.1
Peanuts	1.0
Squid	1.0
Almonds	1.0
Curry powder	1.0
Pistachio nuts, roasted, salted	0.8
Quorn myco-protein	0.8
Currants	0.8
Peanut butter	0.7
Tempeh	0.7
Mushrooms	0.7
Peaches, dried	0.6

RECIPE Fill a sesame seed wholemeal roll with tempeh. Marinate tempeh pieces with a little dressing made by mixing balsamic vinegar, sunflower oil, crushed garlic and tahini. Season with cracked black pepper. Char-grill and serve with salad greens.

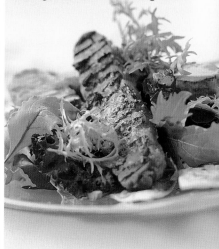

RECIPE Simmer tempeh in a lightly spiced coconut curry with cashew nuts and your choice of vegetables.

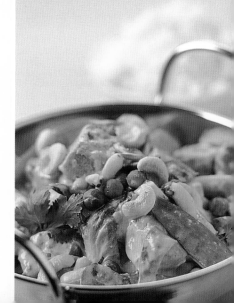

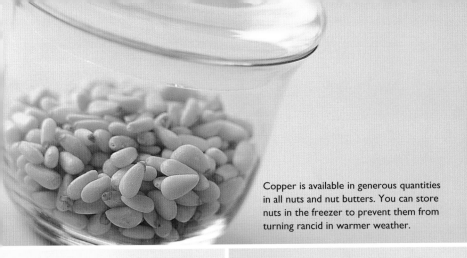

Copper is available in generous quantities in all nuts and nut butters. You can store nuts in the freezer to prevent them from turning rancid in warmer weather.

Oysters are a source of copper, although the levels can vary depending on where they are grown. Cooked oysters have nearly twice as much copper as the raw ones.

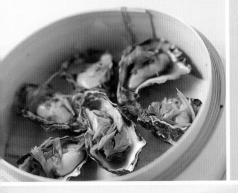

COPPER assists the body in the metabolism of iron and fat. It is required to maintain the heart muscle and tissue and the immune and central nervous systems. Copper is also involved in the formation of melanin and is important for healthy hair and skin. Deficiency is rare, but causes decreased immunity, anaemia, osteoporosis and degeneration of the heart muscle and nervous system.

RECIPE Stir-fry cleaned, honeycombed squid pieces with plenty of crushed garlic, shredded ginger and peanut oil until the squid turns white. Add sliced spring onion and a few generous splashes of sweet chilli sauce and fresh lime.

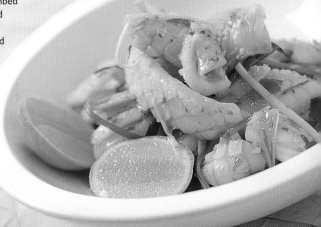

MINERALS – TRACE
MANGANESE

SAFE INTAKE
Adults: more than 1.4 mg/day.

FOOD SOURCES	mg per 100 g
Wheat germ	12.3
Wheat bran	9.0
Pine nuts	7.9
Seaweed, nori, dried	6.0
Macadamia nuts, salted	5.5
Hazelnuts	4.9
Pecan nuts	4.6
Oatmeal	3.7
Mushrooms, oyster	3.6
Crispbread, rye	3.5
Pineapple, dried	3.4
Walnuts	3.4
Muesli, no added sugar	2.6
Sunflower seeds	2.2
Quorn myco-protein	2.1
Peanuts	2.1
Wholemeal bread	1.9
Peanut butter	1.8
Almonds	1.7
Cashew nuts	1.7
Sesame seeds	1.5
Blackberries	1.4
Coconut cream	1.3
Pasta, wholemeal, boiled	0.9
Rice, brown, boiled	0.9
Pineapple, canned in juice	0.9
Watercress	0.6
White bread	0.5
Sweet potato, baked	0.5
Spinach, boiled	0.5
Houmous	0.5
Apples, dried	0.5
Red kidney beans, boiled	0.5
Mussels, canned or bottled	0.5

RECIPE Steam mussels in some white wine with chopped fresh lemon grass and chopped tomato. Mop up the delicious juice with wholemeal bread.

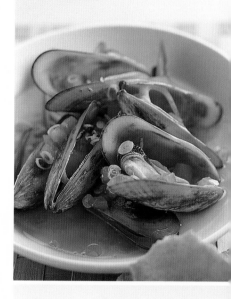

RECIPE For a delicious milkshake, process blackberries, wheat germ, hazelnuts, coconut cream and milk in a blender.

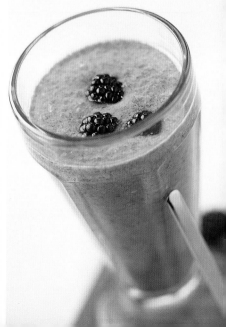

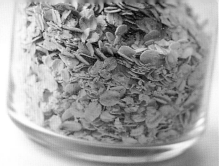

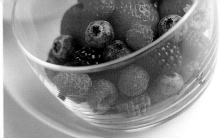

Although manganese occurs naturally in whole grains and cereals, up to 90 per cent can be removed in the milling process, so choose whole grains that have not been subjected to unnecessary amounts of processing.

Add manganese to your diet by snacking on fresh berries in season. Mixed with ice and a little fruit juice, they make a refreshing summer drink.

Good dietary sources are nuts, seeds and wholegrain cereals. Make up a nut and seed praline that can be eaten as a snack or crumbled and served over ice cream.

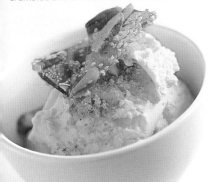

MANGANESE has quite a varied role in the body. It has been found to be an effective antioxidant. It is necessary for the formation of bone and sex hormones and is also involved in carbohydrate and fat metabolism, as well as proper brain functioning. Deficiency is rare and unlikely in normal circumstances.

Large quantities of manganese can be found in all types of seaweed. To add manganese to the diet, try sprinkling shredded roasted seaweed (nori) on rice or salads.

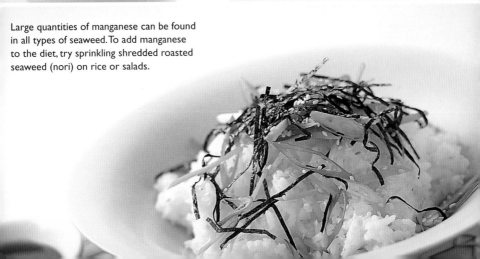

MINERALS – TRACE
IODINE

REFERENCE NUTRIENT INTAKE
Women and men: 140 mcg/day.
Exact figures for iodine in foods are difficult to
establish but good food sources are listed below.

Seafood and deep-water fish such as cod,
halibut, salmon and haddock are excellent
sources of this mineral. Plant foods grown
in soil by the sea absorb iodine from the
sea spray.

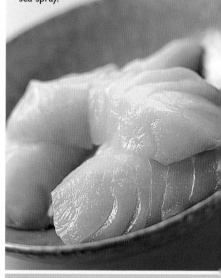

FOOD SOURCES

Bread

Butter

Peppers (capsicum), green

Cereals

Cheese, Cheddar

Clams

Cod

Cottage cheese

Crab

Cream

Dairy products

Eggs

Fruits

Haddock

Lettuce

Lobster

Meat

Milk

Mussels

Oysters

Peanuts

Pineapple

Prawns

Raisins

Salmon

Salt, iodised

Sardines

Seaweed

Spinach

Tuna, canned

Vegetables

RECIPE Coat salmon fillets in sesame seeds,
wrap with a wide strip of roasted nori and
brush the edges lightly to seal. Pan-fry
until tender and serve with steamed rice
and mayonnaise.

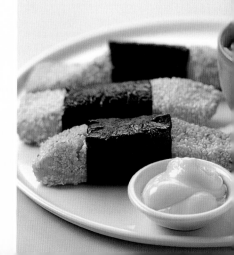

If fish doesn't appeal, you can get iodine from chunks of juicy fresh pineapple, mixed with strawberries and scattered with toasted coconut. Serve with honey and cottage cheese with raisins.

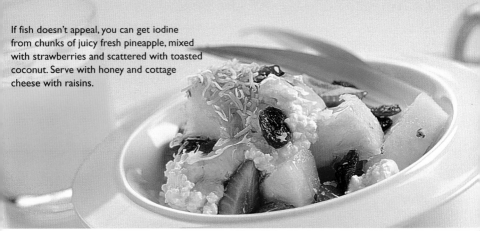

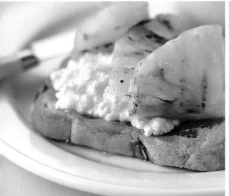

RECIPE Fruit bread topped with sweetened cottage cheese and fried slices of pineapple.

IODINE is essential for the production of the hormones produced by the thyroid gland, which regulate the body's metabolic rate, growth and development, and promote protein synthesis. Selenium is also needed for the synthesis of the thyroid hormones.

Because iodine levels in the soil in some regions are low, iodine is added to salt and is sold as iodised salt. If you have a low-salt diet you may need to monitor your iodine requirements. Deficiency is rare in Western societies because of the relatively high intake of salt.

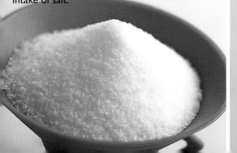

DEFICIENCY Rare in Western societies, deficiency reduces thyroid hormone production and leads to a lowered metabolic rate, which leads to tiredness and weight gain and the thyroid gland becoming enlarged (goitre). If iodine is deficient in pregnancy, there is a greater risk of stillbirth and miscarriage and of mental retardation and growth failure in the baby.

CAUTION Excessive intake of iodine (30 times the RNI) may result in mouth sores, swollen salivary glands, diarrhoea, vomiting, headaches and difficulty breathing. It can lead to goitre, although goitre is more common if the body is iodine deficient.

MINERALS – TRACE
CHROMIUM

SAFE INTAKE
Adults: more than 25 mcg/day.

FOOD SOURCES	mcg per 100 g*
Egg yolk	183
Brewer's yeast	112
Beef	57
Cheese, Cheddar	56
Liver, all types	55
Wine, white/red	45
Bread, wholegrain	42
Black pepper	35
Bread, rye	30
Chilli	30
Apple peel	27
Potatoes, old	27
Oysters	26
Potatoes, new	21
Margarine	18
Spaghetti	15
Spirits	14
Butter	13
Spinach	10
Egg white	8
Oranges	5
Beer	3–30
Apple, peeled	1

Elderly people with diets high in refined foods may be in danger of becoming deficient in chromium because chromium is lost during the milling of grains. Eat wholegrain instead of white bread and use wholemeal flour instead of white.

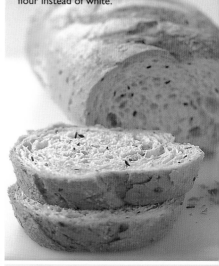

RECIPE Toss cooked spaghetti with shredded fresh spinach, chopped chilli, cracked pepper, toasted wholemeal breadcrumbs and butter.

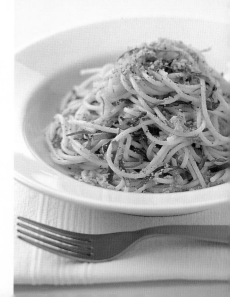

*Australian values.

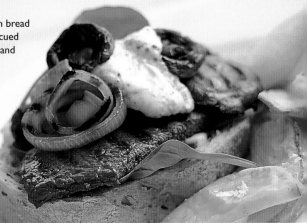

RECIPE Serve thick slices of wholegrain bread topped with baby spinach leaves, barbecued thin beef steaks and barbecued onions and mushrooms. Top with a dollop of sour cream flavoured with honey mustard. Serve with potato wedges.

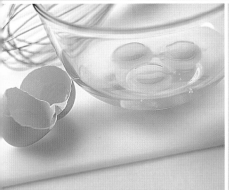

RECIPE For delicious scrambled eggs, whisk some eggs, add plenty of grated Cheddar and cook the mixture in melted butter. Spinach is an ideal accompaniment.

CHROMIUM is essential for the hormone, insulin, to function properly, and is therefore involved in maintaining blood sugar levels. Deficiency is uncommon, but can occur in undernourished elderly people and children with very poor diets. Symptoms include high blood glucose and insulin levels and possibly high blood cholesterol and triglyceride levels.

If you cook with stainless steel cookware, the chromium from the steel is leached into the food and therefore your chromium intake is increased.

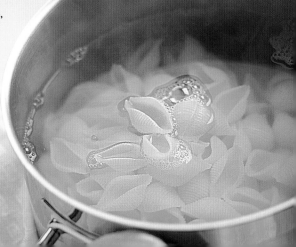

MOLYBDENUM

SAFE INTAKE
Adults: 50–400 mcg/day.
Exact figures for molybdenum are difficult to
establish; listed below are good food sources.

FOOD SOURCES

Apricots

Barley

Beef

Bread, rye

Bread, wholemeal

Cabbage

Carrots

Cauliflower

Cereal grains

Cheese

Chicken

Coconut

Corn

Crab

Eggs

Garlic

Kidneys

Lamb

Legumes

Lentils

Liver, all types

Melon, cantaloupe-type

Milk

Oats, rolled

Onion

Peas, green

Potatoes

Raisins

Rice, brown

Spinach

Sunflower seeds

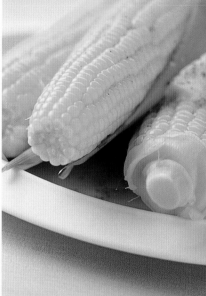

A cob of corn with some butter melted
over the top served with your evening
meal is a simple and tasty way to add
some molybdenum to your diet.

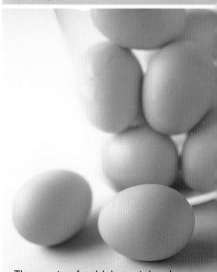

The quantity of molybdenum is largely
dependent on the amount occurring in the
soil that foods are grown in. Processing can
also reduce molybdenum in foods. Eggs are
less susceptible to soil variation and the diets
of chickens are regularly monitored.

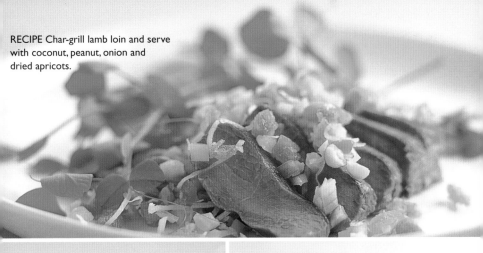

RECIPE Char-grill lamb loin and serve with coconut, peanut, onion and dried apricots.

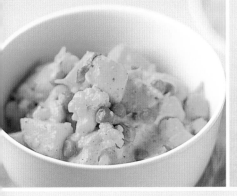

A potato, pea and cauliflower curry in coconut milk, served with brown rice is a good way of adding molybdenum to the diet.

MOLYBDENUM is necessary to activate certain major enzymes in the body. These enzymes are needed for DNA synthesis and for the production of uric acid. Molybdenum is also important for the production of waste products so they can be excreted from the body. Deficiency is rare and unlikely to occur under normal conditions.

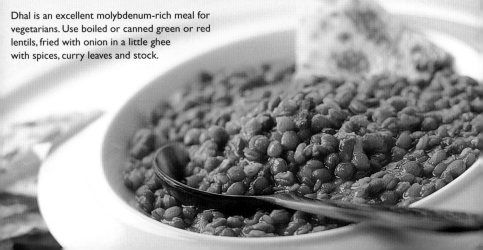

Dhal is an excellent molybdenum-rich meal for vegetarians. Use boiled or canned green or red lentils, fried with onion in a little ghee with spices, curry leaves and stock.

MINERALS – TRACE
FLUORIDE

No RNI or safe intake for adults.
Fluoride figures are difficult to establish but foods containing fluoride are listed below.

FOOD SOURCES

Apples
Asparagus
Barley
Beetroot
Cabbage
Cheese, Cheddar
Corn
Fish, fresh
Fish, canned
Fruits, citrus
Garlic
Kale
Milk, goat's
Milk, skimmed
Millet
Oats
Rice
Rice bran
Salt, sea
Seafood
Spinach
Tea
Water, fluoridated
Watercress

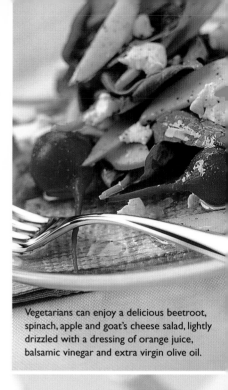

Vegetarians can enjoy a delicious beetroot, spinach, apple and goat's cheese salad, lightly drizzled with a dressing of orange juice, balsamic vinegar and extra virgin olive oil.

Tea can contribute significantly to a person's fluoride intake if they drink a lot, depending on the amount of dry leaves used, brewing time and the fluoride content in the water.

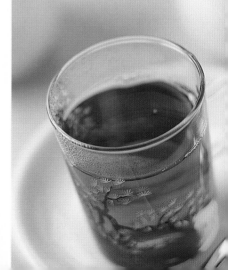

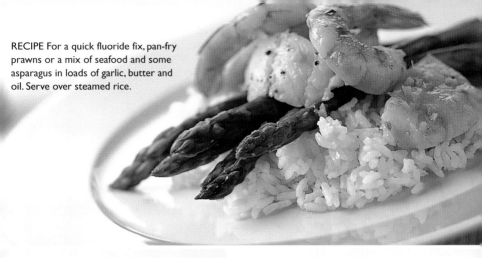

RECIPE For a quick fluoride fix, pan-fry prawns or a mix of seafood and some asparagus in loads of garlic, butter and oil. Serve over steamed rice.

People who choose not to drink water containing fluoride can obtain the mineral by incorporating seafood in their diet.

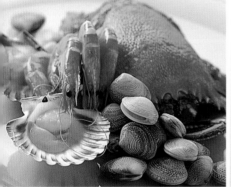

FLUORIDE is contained in every bone in our bodies as well as teeth. It reduces our chances of tooth decay and discolouration. This is why it is added to toothpaste and drinking water. Fluoride may also keep our bones strong. Some people believe that fluoridated water causes health problems, but these claims are not supported by any evidence.

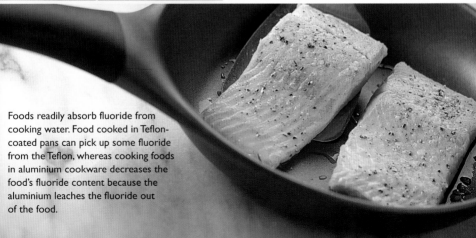

Foods readily absorb fluoride from cooking water. Food cooked in Teflon-coated pans can pick up some fluoride from the Teflon, whereas cooking foods in aluminium cookware decreases the food's fluoride content because the aluminium leaches the fluoride out of the food.

MINERALS – TRACE
SELENIUM

REFERENCE NUTRIENT INTAKE
Women: 60 mcg/day. (Lactation: 75 mcg/day.)
Men: 75mcg/day.

FOOD SOURCES	mcg per 100 g
Brazil nuts	1530
Kidney, pig, fried	270
Mixed nuts and raisins	170
Lobster, boiled	130
Tuna, canned in oil	90
Kidney, lamb, fried	88
Lemon sole, steamed	73
Squid	66
Mullet, red, grilled	54
Scallops, steamed	51
Sardines, canned in oil	49
Sunflower seeds	49
Herring, grilled	46
Shrimps, boiled	46
Plaice, grilled	45
Mussels, boiled	43
Kipper, baked	43
Mackerel, canned in brine	42
Wholemeal bread	35
Cod, baked	34
Salmon, grilled	31
Scone, wholemeal, fruit	31
Crumpets	24
Prawns, boiled	23
Houmous	23
Oysters	23
Pork fillet, lean, grilled	21
Egg yolk	20
Crab, boiled	17
Chicken breast, grilled, no skin	16
Cheese, Cheddar,	12
Eggs, fried	12

Brazil nuts are right at the top of the list as a source of selenium. Eat them as a snack or chop some and serve over your favourite ice cream.

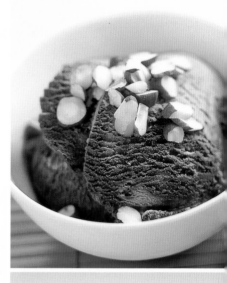

RECIPE Wholemeal bread sandwiches for children, spread with hummus and topped with canned tuna and salad greens, will ensure their selenium requirements are met.

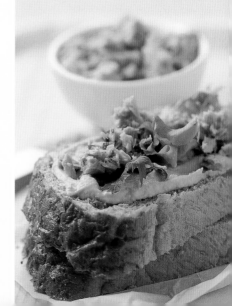

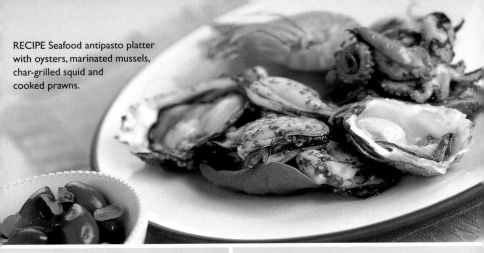

RECIPE Seafood antipasto platter with oysters, marinated mussels, char-grilled squid and cooked prawns.

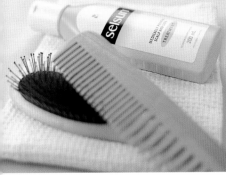

Selenium is easily absorbed through the skin and selenium-based shampoos are extremely effective in the treatment of dandruff or dry scalp.

SELENIUM is best known for its antioxidant properties and works with vitamin E to protect the body against free radicals. Selenium is also essential for the production of thyroid hormones that regulate the metabolic rate in our bodies and may help protect us from heart disease. Selenium deficiency is rare. Do not take daily supplements that contain more than 200 mcg. Toxic symptoms include nervousness, depression, nausea, vomiting and loss of hair and fingernails.

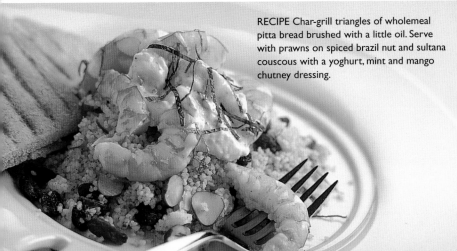

RECIPE Char-grill triangles of wholemeal pitta bread brushed with a little oil. Serve with prawns on spiced brazil nut and sultana couscous with a yoghurt, mint and mango chutney dressing.

FOOD JOURNAL

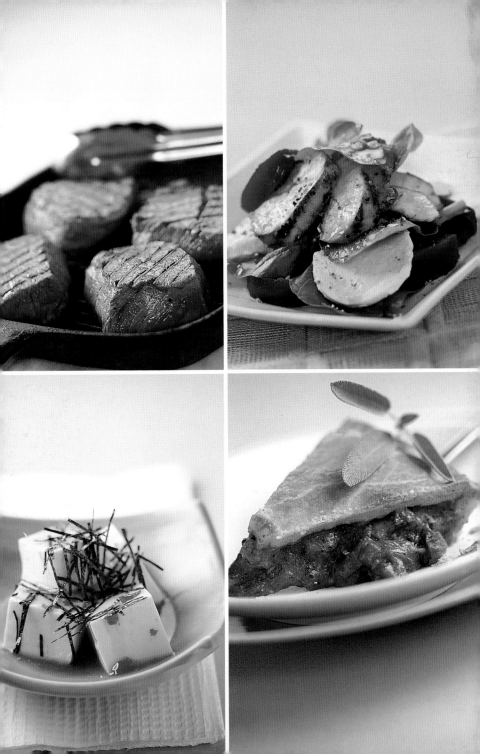

FOOD JOURNAL

A food journal is an excellent way of keeping an accurate record of what you eat. If you fill it in honestly and regularly it will highlight areas of your diet which can be improved. If you also keep a note of whom you ate with, how you felt and how much exercise you take, the journal can become more than a list of meals—it can develop into a scientific document that will help any health professional give you better nutritional advice.

Choose a "normal" week to start filling in your journal. If you are about to go on holiday, or have visitors then it is better to wait for a few weeks until you start. Fill in the journal as you go through the day. If you wait until several days have elapsed before filling in the gaps you will almost certainly make an error which will mean that the journal is not accurate.

WHAT DID I EAT?
What did you eat? Be sure to include everything. Dressings, condiments and sauces can all contribute to your eating patterns. Remember to include all snacks and drinks.

HOW MUCH DID I EAT?
You need to keep a close watch on the amount of food you consume. Estimate the size (in millimetres/inches), the volume (in fl/oz /cups), the weight, and the quantity for each item.

WHEN DID I EAT?
Enter the time at which you ate. Time is often one of the more important aspects of healthy eating so try to be as accurate as possible.

Photocopy the following pages to create your own monthly food journal.

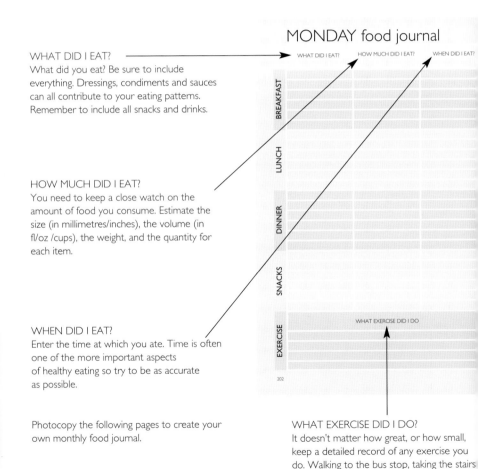

MONDAY food journal

WHAT EXERCISE DID I DO?
It doesn't matter how great, or how small, keep a detailed record of any exercise you do. Walking to the bus stop, taking the stairs anything that increases your heart rate will influence the number of calories your body is burning.

It is hard but be honest and include everything. You will gain nothing by pretending that you didn't eat certain foods!

When you have kept a journal for a month, you will be able to see patterns emerging that will suggest how you may improve your eating, and lifestyle, habits. It may become clear that you only eat chocolate when you are feeling depressed, or only eat ice-cream when watching late-night television. Knowing that these connections exist will help you to monitor and change them.

WHERE / WITH WHOM DID I EAT?

WHAT WAS I DOING?

WHAT MOOD WAS I IN?

HOW MANY CALORIES HAVE I CONSUMED?

HOW MANY CALORIES DID I BURN?

WHERE / WITH WHOM DID I EAT?
Our eating habits are frequently affected by where we eat and how many people are with us. By filling in this part of the journal we can easily see the effects that eating in a group, or eating out of doors has on us.

WHAT WAS I DOING?
We often find ourselves eating while reading, talking, walking, watching television or even travelling to work. Make a note of exactly what you were doing while you were eating to see if certain patterns emerge.

WHAT MOOD WAS I IN?
The areas of the brain that regulate our emotional responses are interconnected with the parts of the brain that regulate our eating patterns. As a result, there is a direct connection between how we feel and what we eat. Use this column of the journal to record your feelings and see if anxiety, stress, happiness or sadness are reflected in the types of food you eat.

HOW MANY CALORIES DID I BURN?
Keep an accurate record of the amount of exercise you take each day. Physical activity is the best way to burn-off calories and twenty minutes of the following popular activities will use up the calories shown. Dancing 120; cycling 160; running 90; aerobics 140; weights 140; cleaning 50; driving 35; swimming 100; tennis 120; rowing 200; golf 45; circuit training 260; skipping 100; gardening 160 and skiing 130 calories.

HOW MANY CALORIES HAVE I CONSUMED?
Use the tables in this book to estimate your calorie intake for the day. Be as precise as you can. Use the table on page 12 to work out how many calories you should be consuming daily.

SUNDAY food journal

	WHAT DID I EAT?	HOW MUCH DID I EAT?	WHEN DID I EAT?
BREAKFAST			
LUNCH			
DINNER			
SNACKS			

	WHAT EXERCISE DID I DO
EXERCISE	

WHERE / WITH WHOM DID I EAT?	WHAT WAS I DOING?	WHAT MOOD WAS I IN?

HOW MANY CALORIES HAVE I CONSUMED?	HOW MANY CALORIES DID I BURN?

MONDAY food journal

	WHAT DID I EAT?	HOW MUCH DID I EAT?	WHEN DID I EAT?
BREAKFAST			
LUNCH			
DINNER			
SNACKS			

EXERCISE	WHAT EXERCISE DID I DO

WHERE / WITH WHOM DID I EAT?	WHAT WAS I DOING?	WHAT MOOD WAS I IN?

HOW MANY CALORIES HAVE I CONSUMED?	HOW MANY CALORIES DID I BURN?

TUESDAY food journal

	WHAT DID I EAT?	HOW MUCH DID I EAT?	WHEN DID I EAT?
BREAKFAST			
LUNCH			
DINNER			
SNACKS			

EXERCISE — WHAT EXERCISE DID I DO

WHERE / WITH WHOM DID I EAT?	WHAT WAS I DOING?	WHAT MOOD WAS I IN?

HOW MANY CALORIES HAVE I CONSUMED?	HOW MANY CALORIES DID I BURN?

WEDNESDAY food journal

	WHAT DID I EAT?	HOW MUCH DID I EAT?	WHEN DID I EAT?
BREAKFAST			
LUNCH			
DINNER			
SNACKS			

EXERCISE	WHAT EXERCISE DID I DO

WHERE / WITH WHOM DID I EAT?	WHAT WAS I DOING?	WHAT MOOD WAS I IN?

HOW MANY CALORIES HAVE I CONSUMED?	HOW MANY CALORIES DID I BURN?

THURSDAY food journal

	WHAT DID I EAT?	HOW MUCH DID I EAT?	WHEN DID I EAT?
BREAKFAST			
LUNCH			
DINNER			
SNACKS			

EXERCISE

WHAT EXERCISE DID I DO

WHERE / WITH WHOM DID I EAT?	WHAT WAS I DOING?	WHAT MOOD WAS I IN?

HOW MANY CALORIES HAVE I CONSUMED?	HOW MANY CALORIES DID I BURN?

FRIDAY food journal

	WHAT DID I EAT?	HOW MUCH DID I EAT?	WHEN DID I EAT?
BREAKFAST			
LUNCH			
DINNER			
SNACKS			

	WHAT EXERCISE DID I DO	
EXERCISE		

WHERE / WITH WHOM DID I EAT?	WHAT WAS I DOING?	WHAT MOOD WAS I IN?

HOW MANY CALORIES HAVE I CONSUMED?	HOW MANY CALORIES DID I BURN?

SATURDAY food journal

	WHAT DID I EAT?	HOW MUCH DID I EAT?	WHEN DID I EAT?
BREAKFAST			
LUNCH			
DINNER			
SNACKS			

EXERCISE	WHAT EXERCISE DID I DO

WHERE / WITH WHOM DID I EAT?	WHAT WAS I DOING?	WHAT MOOD WAS I IN?

HOW MANY CALORIES HAVE I CONSUMED?	HOW MANY CALORIES DID I BURN?

FOOD TERMS

ABSORPTION is the process whereby nutrients from digested foods are transferred from the gastro-intestinal tract into the bloodstream or lymph system for transport to the body's cells.

ALCOHOL content of different drinks can be measured in units. A unit is equivalent to about 8g or 10ml of pure alcohol. There is approximately 1 unit of alcohol in each of the following:
- 285ml ordinary strength beer, lager or cider;
- a single 25ml measure of spirits;
- a small glass (100ml) of wine or sherry;
- a measure of vermouth or aperitif.

Some research suggests that middle-aged and older people who drink small amounts of alcohol on a regular basis appear to be at lower risk of heart disease than non-drinkers. Alcohol may have a protective effect on the heart in two ways – it directly affects the amount of cholesterol carried by the blood and it reduces the likelihood of blood clotting. However, these beneficial effects only appear to apply to men over 40 and postmenopausal women who drink no more than 2 and 1 units a day, respectively. There is no evidence of these beneficial effects in younger people, nor any special benefit from specific drinks (for example, red wine). At intakes of more than three standard drinks a day, alcohol has adverse effects on blood pressure, increases the risk of stroke, cancer and weight gain. Government guidelines recommend that men drink no more than three standard drinks a day and women no more than two standard drink a day for good health, with some alcohol-free days each week. It's important to know that alcohol is second only to fat in its energy content (29kJ/g) and regular drinking may cause weight gain and nutrient deficiencies.

ANTIOXIDANTS such as vitamins C, E and beta carotene (pre-vitamin A found in fruit and vegetables) are powerful, protective substances that mop up potentially harmful molecules called free radicals. These free radicals are produced during normal bodily processes, but their production can be increased by a high fat diet and environmental pollution, such as cigarette smoke and exhaust fumes. If too many free radicals are formed in the body, they may contribute to the development of diseases such as cancer and heart disease. The best way of getting the right mixture and balance of antioxidants is to regularly eat a wide variety of fruit, vegetables and wholegrain foods. Antioxidant supplements do not appear to have the same health benefits as foods naturally rich in antioxidants. In fact, there is some evidence that beta carotene supplements have no protective effect at best and may even increase rates of lung cancer at worst. Beta carotene supplements should therefore be avoided as a means of protecting against cancer, whereas a healthy diet and lifestyle will benefit your current and future health. Other high-dose, purified supplements should also be used with caution because they cannot be assumed to be without risk. Always seek medical advice before taking any vitamin or mineral supplements.

BLOOD GLUCOSE is the amount of sugar (glucose) circulating in the bloodstream. It is an energy source for the brain, muscles and every cell in the body.

BLOOD PRESSURE is the pressure of the blood in the arteries as the heart pumps it around the body. High blood pressure (hyper-tension) increases the risk of heart disease. When the heart contracts (systolic pressure) the 'normal' pressure is less than 130mm mercury (Hg). When the heart relaxes (diastolic pressure) before the next beat, the 'normal' pressure is less than 85 Hg (written as 130/85). A blood pressure reading between 130/85 and 140/90 is classified as mild hypertension and a reading higher than 180/110 is severe HT. Blood pressure tends to rise gradually with age so that the average blood pressure of a 65-year-old is 160/90. Reducing salt intake, quitting smoking, getting regular physical activity, limiting alcohol intake and maintaining a healthy weight can help lower blood pressure.

CALORIES (see KILOJOULES)

CARBOHYDRATES are a major source of energy in the diet and should make up at least 55% of the kilojoules we eat. There are three main types of carbohydrate: starches, sugars and fibre. The sugars and starches are digested into sugar in the body, which is the body's main fuel or energy source.

Sugars can be divided into different types:
1. Non-milk extrinsic sugars (NMEs) are those not contained within the cellular structure of food, such as 'added' sugar in drinks, confectionery, spreads, breakfast cereals, cakes and biscuits. Official healthy eating guidelines state that no more than 11% of the kilojoules we eat should come from NME's, but the average intake is about 14%.
2. Milk sugars (lactose) are those found in milk and therefore dairy products.
3. Intrinsic sugars are those that are an integral part of the cell structure, such as the sugar in fruit and vegetables.

CHOLESTEROL is a type of fat found in animals. It is not essential to eat foods containing cholesterol because it is made in the body by the liver and carried around in the blood by lipoproteins. A high blood cholesterol level can result in cholesterol building up inside the arteries, which is a major risk factor for heart disease. Surprisingly, the saturated fat in foods is more likely to increase blood cholesterol than dietary cholesterol (the cholesterol found in foods of animal origin). Reducing your saturated fat intake as part of a healthy diet can help lower a raised blood cholesterol level.

COENZYMES are small non-protein molecules that bind to enzymes and allow them to function normally by acting as carriers of atoms or electrons in metabolic reactions.

DENTAL CARIES (tooth decay) is the progressive destruction of teeth by acid generated by the bacteria in plaque on the surfaces of the teeth. The bacteria produce acid as a by-product of the metabolism of dietary carbohydrates and the plaque holds the acid in contact with the tooth like a piece of blotting paper. If sticky (high in added sugars), sugary or starchy foods, such as toffees or soft white bread, are eaten too often, acid levels remain high and tooth decay is likely.

DIABETES MELLITUS is a disease whose incidence is rapidly growing in western societies, in which carbohydrate metabolism is impaired due to the insufficient production of insulin or the inability of cells to respond to insulin. If not controlled, it results in elevated blood glucose and cholesterol levels and is associated with an increased risk of heart disease.

DIGESTION is the process of breaking down nutrients in foods to small molecules that can be absorbed into the bloodstream and lymph system and then carried to the body's cells. Food digestion involves both mechanical (chewing, mixing) and chemical (enzymes and digestive juices) processes.

ELECTROLYTES are electrically charged particles that separate in water to form positively or negatively charged ions (eg. sodium, potassium, chloride). They are required for the regulation of normal fluid balance in cells, the entry of nutrients into cells, and are needed for nerves and muscles to function.

ENERGY is required for all bodily processes and physical and mental activity. Energy is obtained from the metabolism of carbohydrates, proteins, fats and alcohol. Vitamins and minerals do not directly provide energy, but are required for the metabolic processes that obtain the energy in the other nutrients. Energy is measured in either kilojoules (kJ) or kilo-calories (referred to as Calories). One Calorie = 4.2 kJ.

ENZYMES are protein molecules that catalyse metabolic reactions, allowing the reactions to occur without being used or changed themselves. There are thousands of enzymes in the body, all essential for normal functioning and health. Some inherited diseases are due to the absence or impaired action of only one enzyme.

ESSENTIAL FATTY ACIDS are fatty acids that must be obtained from foods because they can't be made in the body at all or in sufficient quantities. Linoleic acid, an omega-6 polyunsaturated fatty acid, and alpha-linolenic acid, an omega-3 polyunsaturated fatty acid, are essential fatty acids. They are needed for healthy skin, wound healing, and good vision and hearing, and can be used to make other types of fatty acids needed in the body. Omega-3 fats are found mainly in oily fish, whereas omega-6 fats are present in vegetable oils and nuts.

FIBRE Fibre is also known as non-starch polysaccharides. See *separate listing.*

FLAVONOIDS are antioxidant compounds that give colour to flowers, fruit and vegetables. They have been shown to reduce blood clotting and LDL-cholesterol oxidation (involved in the process of heart disease).

FREE RADICALS are highly reactive unstable molecules formed during the normal metabolic processes in the body. They cause damage to cells and play a role in the development of diseases such as cancer, arthritis and heart disease. Antioxidants are thought to 'mop up' free radicals, preventing them from doing harm.

HEART DISEASE and strokes are jointly referred to as 'cardiovascular disease'. Symptoms of heart disease include angina (pains in the arms and/or chest) and poor blood flow in the limbs. Strokes are usually caused by clots in blood vessels that supply blood to the brain. The probability of someone suffering from cardiovascular disease is determined by a number of risk factors including age, sex, family history, blood pressure, the level of blood cholesterol, triglycerides and sugar, obesity, diabetes, smoking, ethnic group, stress and physical activity level. Many of these risk factors can be controlled by a healthy, low-fat diet and getting regular exercise.

INSULIN is a hormone produced by the pancreas. It is essential for preventing the blood sugar level from rising too high after eating. Insulin stimulates the uptake of glucose from the blood into cells for use as energy or storage and the uptake and storage of fat and the uptake and metabolism of amino acids from the blood.

KILOJOULES are a measure of energy (for example, the energy in food and the amount of energy our bodies need). KJ is an abbreviation for kilojoules, which is the metric equivalent of

calories. Kcals or Cals are abbreviations for kilocalories and these are what most people know as calories. Most nutrition labels show figures for both Cals and kJs. There are approximately 4.2kJ in 1Cal, which is why kJ values are always higher.

METABOLISM is the chemical processes occurring in the body by which nutrients are converted into energy.

MINERALS are nutrients in foods needed in small amounts for important bodily processes such as maintaining the body's fluid balance and the structure of hormones, bones, and teeth, the regulation of blood pressure, wound healing, and the activity of muscles and nerves. Minerals can't be made in the body, so we have to obtain them from our diet. There are two classes of minerals and these are explained on page 108.

MONOUNSATURATED FAT is one of the three main types of fat found in foods. Foods containing a high proportion of mono-unsaturated fat include olive, canola and fish oils, macadamia nuts, avocados and some meats. Replacing saturated fat in the diet with monounsaturated fat, as part of a low-fat diet, can help lower a high blood cholesterol level and reduce the risk of heart disease.

NEUROTRANSMITTERS are a chemical produced by a nerve cell that can stimulate or inhibit the activity of another nerve.

NON-STARCH POLYSACCHARIDES is the technical name for dietary fibre. It includes soluble and insoluble fibre. Soluble fibre can be found in oats, pulses, barley and fruits and vegetables. It may help lower a high blood cholesterol level if consumed as part of a healthy low-fat diet. Insoluble fibre is the type of fibre found in grain and grain products (bread, pasta, breakfast cereals, rice), especially wholegrain varieties. It can prevent constipation and reduce the risk of other bowel problems such as haemorrhoids and bowel cancer. High fibre foods tend to be low in fat and have the added bonus of filling you up while providing relatively few kilojoules. Healthy eating guidelines recommend that we eat 30g of fibre each day. However, many people eat less than 15g a day.

NUTRIENTS are chemicals in foods that provide energy, contribute to growth, repair and structure and help metabolic processes. Proteins, carbohydrates, fats, vitamins, minerals and water are all classified as nutrients.

OMEGA-3 FATTY ACIDS are one type of essential polyunsaturated fatty acids that tend to be lacking in Western diets. Omega-3 fats can be found in oily fish (salmon, tuna, mackerel, trout), fish oils, linseeds and linseed oil, walnuts and omega-3-enriched hen's eggs. There is evidence to suggest that consuming these fatty acids by eating oily fish (herring, mackerel, trout, salmon) at least three to four times a week can help reduce the risk of blood clots and heart attacks. These fish oils help reduce inflammation, which may be of benefit to people with arthritis.

OSTEOPOROSIS is sometimes called 'brittle bone disease' and results in overly fragile, weak bones that fracture very easily. Up until early adulthood, our bones grow in length and also become more dense as more calcium and other minerals are deposited in them. This makes them strong and growth continues until our early 30's when bone density reaches its peak. From then on, bones become thinner as we get older as a normal part of ageing. Excessive bone loss (osteoporosis) can be prevented by regularly eating plenty of calcium-rich foods, getting regular weight-bearing exercise, not smoking and only drinking alcohol in moderation.

PHYTATE is a phosphorus-containing compound found in seeds, nuts and grains. It can bind minerals and prevent them from being absorbed.

PHYTOESTROGENS are natural oestrogen-like substances found in plant-based foods. Wholebean soya products are an excellent source of phytoestrogens in the diet. Some studies have suggested that diets high in phytoestrogens are associated with low rates of breast cancer. However, as yet there is insufficient evidence to prove this.

POLYUNSATURATED FAT is one of the three main types of fats found in foods. It can be divided into two groups known as omega-6 and omega-3 polyunsaturated fats according to their structure. The omega-6 polyunsaturated fats are the main type of fat in most vegetable oils (sunflower, corn and soy bean), nuts and seeds. Replacing saturated fats with polyunsaturated, as part of a low-fat diet, can help reduce a high blood LDL-cholesterol level. By making sure that you don't eat omega-6 fats exclusively (and very little omega-3), you can prevent the level of 'good' HDL-cholesterol from falling as well.

PRESERVATIVES are substances added to food to prevent spoilage and extend shelf life by retarding chemical, physical and microbial changes in food.

PROTEIN is needed in the diet to provide structural material for the growth and repair of tissues. Proteins are also an energy source, and if more protein is consumed than the body needs, the extra is burnt off or converted into sugar for fuel or fat for storage. Proteins are large molecules made up of small units called amino acids. When proteins are eaten, they are digested or broken down into their constituent amino acids, which are then absorbed. The body can then use them to make its own new proteins, including enzymes, hormones and the nerves' chemical messengers (neuro-transmitters). There are 20 different amino acids found in plant and animal proteins, but the body has a limited capacity to convert one amino acid into another. Some amino acids cannot be made from others and have to be obtained from the diet. These are called essential amino acids. Proteins in animal foods, such as eggs, meat and milk, contain all the essential amino acids needed by the body and are therefore called complete or high-quality proteins. Proteins in plant foods, such as cereals and beans, don't contain all of the essential amino acids and are therefore called incomplete proteins. However, it's possible to get complete protein by combining different plant foods, such as legumes and grains, or adding some dairy foods. When eaten together (eg. beans on toast) the protein 'quality' is as good as foods of animal origin. For most people, protein quality is not worth worrying about, because most eat more than they need. Children given a vegetarian diet need a good mix of plant proteins to give them the high-quality protein they need for growth and development. The recommended daily intake of protein for adults is 0.75–1g of protein per kilogram of body weight. This equates to at least 45g per day for women and 55g per day for men.

PRO-VITAMIN is a compound that can be converted into the active form of a vitamin in the body.

RECOMMENDED DIETARY INTAKE (RDI) VALUES In many countries, committees of health experts have reviewed all the scientific evidence regarding the amounts of vitamins and minerals needed to prevent deficiency and promote good health. Using this data, the experts have calculated recommended dietary intake (RDI) values for some nutrients, which are the amounts needed daily to prevent deficiency in practically all healthy people. In the table below, the RDIs for various nutrients are given in milligrams (mg) or micrograms (mcg). These RDI values actually exceed the needs of most people, because they contain a safety margin to cover people who are less efficient in absorbing vitamins and minerals or who need greater amounts. Therefore, if a person's intake of a nutrient is less than the RDI they may not necessarily be deficient. Over a long period of time, relatively low intakes could lead to deficiency, but this would need to be confirmed by medical tests.

SATURATED FAT is one of the three main types of fat in foods. A high proportion of saturated fats can be found in foods such as full-fat milk and dairy products, fatty meat and meat products, spreads, solid cooking fats, biscuits, cakes and pastries. High intake of saturated fat can increase the blood cholesterol level and therefore the risk of heart disease. According to current healthy eating guidelines, saturated fat should provide no more than 10% of the kilojoules we eat. Choosing low-fat dairy products and lean cuts of meat and not eating biscuits and pastries on a regular basis will help lower your saturated fat intake.

SODIUM CHLORIDE is the chemical name for salt. Salt is added to many processed foods, so many people regularly eat more salt than they are aware of and more than they really need. A high salt intake can increase blood pressure and the risk of heart disease. Healthy eating guidelines recommend that we eat less than 6g of salt per day, which is still in excess of physiological requirements. Most people need to cut their salt intake by at least one third to reach this goal. Since most of the salt we eat comes from manufactured foods, it's a good idea to choose reduced-salt products wherever possible. Salt should also not be added to cooking water or sauces or cooked meals. Learn to appreciate the natural flavours of foods without the over-powering taste of salt.

SYNERGIST is a compound that interacts with another to produce increased activity, which is greater than the sum of the effects produced by either compound alone.

TRANS FATTY ACIDS have a slightly different structure to other unsaturated fatty acids and a high intake is thought to have the same undesirable effect of elevating blood cholesterol as saturated fat. Trans fats occur naturally in some foods and are also formed during the process of changing liquid vegetable oils into solid margarines. Since it was discovered that relatively high intakes of trans fats could elevate blood cholesterol, the trans fat content of most margarines has been reduced. It is recommended that no more than 2% of the kilojoules we eat should come from trans fats.

VITAMINS are nutrients that are only needed in small amounts but have powerful effects. They are required for the normal functioning of every organ and for many important processes such as growth, reproduction and tissue repair. Although vitamins themselves are not a source of energy, they are needed to liberate the energy from dietary carbohydrate, protein, fat and alcohol for the body's cells to use. There are two classes of vitamin: fat-soluble and water-soluble and these are described in detail on page 108.

USEFUL INFORMATION

The recipes in this book were developed using a tablespoon measure of 20 ml. In some other countries the tablespoon is 15 ml. For most recipes this difference will not be noticeable but, for recipes using baking powder, gelatine, bicarbonate of soda, small amounts of flour and cornflour, we suggest that, if you are using the smaller tablespoon, you add an extra teaspoon for each tablespoon.

The recipes in this book are written using convenient cup measurements. You can buy special measuring cups in the supermarket or use an ordinary household cup: first you need to check it holds 250 ml (8 fl oz) by filling it with water and measuring the water (pour it into a measuring jug or a carton that you know holds 250 ml). This cup can then be used for both liquid and dry cup measurements.

Liquid cup measures

1/4 cup	60 ml	2 fluid oz
1/3 cup	80 ml	2 3/4 fluid oz
1/2 cup	125 ml	4 fluid oz
3/4 cup	180 ml	6 fluid oz
1 cup	250 ml	8 fluid oz

Spoon measures

1/4 teaspoon	1.25 ml
1/2 teaspoon	2.5 ml
1 teaspoon	5 ml
1 tablespoon	20 ml

Nutritional Information

The nutritional information given for each recipe does not include any garnishes or accompaniments, such as rice or pasta, unless they are included in specific quantities in the ingredients list. The nutritional values are approximations and can be affected by biological and seasonal variations in foods, the unknown composition of some manufactured foods and uncertainty in the dietary database. Nutrient data given are derived primarily from the NUTTAB95 database produced by the Australian and New Zealand Food Authority.

Oven Temperatures
You may find cooking times vary depending on the oven you are using. For fan-forced ovens, as a general rule, set oven temperature to 20°C lower than indicated in the recipe.

Note: Those who might be at risk from the effects of salmonella food poisoning (the elderly, pregnant women, young children and those suffering from immune deficiency diseases) should consult their GP with any concerns about eating raw eggs.

Alternative names (UK/US)

bicarbonate of soda	—	baking soda
besan flour	—	chickpea flour
capsicum	—	red or green bell pepper
chickpeas	—	garbanzo beans
cornflour	—	cornstarch
fresh coriander	—	cilantro
single cream	—	cream
aubergine	—	eggplant
flat-leaf parsley	—	Italian parsley
hazelnut	—	filbert
minced beef	—	ground beef
plain flour	—	all-purpose flour
polenta	—	cornmeal
prawn	—	shrimp
Roma tomato	—	plum or egg tomato
sambal oelek	—	chilli paste
mangetout	—	snow pea
spring onion	—	scallion
thick cream	—	heavy cream
tomato purée	—	tomato paste
courgette	—	zucchini

Weight

10 g	1/4 oz	220 g	7 oz	425 g	14 oz
30 g	1 oz	250 g	8 oz	475 g	15 oz
60 g	2 oz	275 g	9 oz	500 g	1 lb
90 g	3 oz	300 g	10 oz	600 g	1 1/4 lb
125 g	4 oz	330 g	11 oz	650 g	1 lb 5 oz
150 g	5 oz	375 g	12 oz	750 g	1 1/2 lb
185 g	6 oz	400 g	13 oz	1 kg	2 lb

Published in 2004 by Bay Books® Australia, a division of
Murdoch Magazines Pty Ltd, Pier 8/9, 23 Hickson Road, Millers Point, NSW 2000
Phone: +61 (2) 4352 7000 Fax: +61 (2) 4352 7026

Nutrition Consultants: Dr Susanna Holt
Text: Dr Susanna Holt, Jody Vassallo, Kay Halsey

Colour separation by Colourscan in Singapore
Printed in China by Midas Printing (Asia) Limited

National Library of Australia
Cataloguing-in-Publication Data

ISBN 1 74045 424 3.

NUTRITION: The nutritional values are approximations and can be affected by biological and seasonal
variations in foods, the unknown composition of some manufactured foods and uncertainty in the
dietary database. Nutrient data given are derived from information provided by manufacturers and the
official NUTTAB95 (Diet 1) nutritional values database produced by the Australian New Zealand
Food Authority. Commonwealth of Australia copyright reproduced by permission.

The figures for RNI in this book relate to adults. The nutritional values of foods are approximations and
can be affected by biological and seasonal variations in foods, the unknown composition of some
manufactured foods and uncertainty in the dietary database. Nutrient values of foods were obtained
from Foodworks, nutrition software by Xyris Software (Australia) Pty. Ltd., based on the Australian Food
Composition Tables database (NUTTAB) from the Australia New Zealand Food Authority (ANZFA).
RNI figures were obtained from Recommended Dietary Intakes for use in Australia,
National Health and Medical Research Council (NHMRC) 1991.

IMPORTANT: This book is intended as a guide for following a healthy diet. Anybody with specific dietary
needs, such as the elderly, pregnant women, young children and those suffering from immune deficiency
diseases, should consult their doctor before changing their diet.